"Paula Freedman-Diamond candidly talks about how her quest for perfection was her way of quieting her inner critic. She shows us how striving for unrealistic standards rooted in racism, misogyny, ableism, and ageism are then promoted by diet, wellness, and hustle cultures. Through tools derived from acceptance and commitment therapy (ACT) and intuitive eating, this valuable book offers a way out of this all-encompassing life toward the freedom that comes with inner trust."

—**Elyse Resch, MS, RDN, CEDS-S**, FAND Nutrition Therapist, coauthor of *Intuitive Eating*, and author of *The Intuitive Eating Workbook for Teens*

"In a personal, practical, and deeply empowering way, Freedman-Diamond helps readers identify the sneaky, quiet ways toxic striving has infiltrated our lives and stolen our joy and power. As she writes, 'This book won't give you answers; it will help you discover your own answers.' She accomplishes her end goal of helping readers find ourselves in the midst of toxic messaging begging us to abandon ourselves in favor of perfection."

—**Lexie Kite, PhD**, coauthor of *More Than a Body*

"*Toxic Striving* provides a wealth of information on how we often fall into patterns that aren't true to who we are or what we want to be. Through relatable stories and reflection questions that spark 'aha' moments of self-awareness and a rekindling of the long-ignored intuition, *Toxic Striving* helps break unhelpful striving patterns, fosters a connection with our values, and guides us in creating an authentic life."

—**Sarah Pegrum, PhD**, psychologist, and author of *Break the Binds of Weight Stigma*

T0182718

"Paula Freedman-Diamond illuminates the connection between wellness culture and productivity culture; by making this important bridge, she is able to guide readers to regain trust in themselves and opt out of toxic striving using practical, evidence-based strategies from ACT and intuitive eating."

—**Alexis Conason, PsyD**, psychologist, and author of
The Diet-Free Revolution

"This is a fun book to read. It is filled with captivating anecdotes and exercises from a handful of empirically supported treatments, including ACT. Anyone struggling with clinical perfectionism, self-judgment, or body-image issues should read from this book and practice what it teaches."

—**Michael P. Twohig, PhD**, professor of psychology at Utah
State University, and coauthor of *The Anxious Perfectionist*

"In this gem of a book, Paula Freedman-Diamond weaves together the intersection of the culture of productivity and perfectionism with diet and wellness culture. Written with warmth and clarity, *Toxic Striving* will give you the tools to explore your true values, honor your needs, and practice self-care from a place of attunement so that you can develop a peaceful relationship with food and live a more authentic and satisfying life. Five stars!"

—**Judith Matz, LCSW**, coauthor of *The Emotional Eating,*
Chronic Dieting, Binge Eating, and Body Image Workbook
and *Beyond a Shadow of a Diet*

TOXIC STRIVING

WHY HUSTLE & WELLNESS CULTURE ARE LEAVING US ANXIOUS, STRESSED & BURNED OUT— & HOW TO BREAK FREE

PAULA FREEDMAN-DIAMOND, PSYD

New Harbinger Publications, Inc.

Publisher's Note

This publication is designed to provide accurate and authoritative information in regard to the subject matter covered. It is sold with the understanding that the publisher is not engaged in rendering psychological, financial, legal, or other professional services. If expert assistance or counseling is needed, the services of a competent professional should be sought.

All case studies in this book are composites. Any resemblance to persons living or dead is unintentional and entirely coincidental.

NEW HARBINGER PUBLICATIONS is a registered trademark of New Harbinger Publications, Inc.

New Harbinger Publications is an employee-owned company.

Copyright © 2024 by Paula Freedman-Diamond
New Harbinger Publications, Inc.
5720 Shattuck Avenue
Oakland, CA 94609
www.newharbinger.com

All Rights Reserved

Cover design by Sara Christian

Acquired by Elizabeth Hollis Hansen

Edited by Kandace Little

Library of Congress Cataloging-in-Publication Data on file

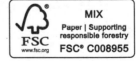

Printed in the United States of America

26		25		24					

| 10 | 9 | 8 | 7 | 6 | 5 | 4 | 3 | 2 | 1 | First Printing |

For my dear friend and partner in toxic-striving recovery,
Sari: Everyone deserves a friend like you.

And for my clients: You have taught me so much about
practicing willingness, vulnerability, and authenticity. It is
an honor and privilege to be part of your journey.

Contents

Foreword   vii

Introduction: The Target Is Always Moving   1

PART 1: *A Job You Didn't Sign Up For*

Chapter 1   How You Were Brainwashed   8

Chapter 2   You Were Never the Problem   22

Chapter 3   How You Learned the Rules   33

Chapter 4   You're Not Special for Drinking Celery Juice   44

PART 2: *Taking Back the Steering Wheel*

Chapter 5   Redefining Your Values   56

Chapter 6   Unconditional Permission to Be Human   67

Chapter 7   Tapping into Your Hunger   78

Chapter 8   Embracing Fullness and Satisfaction   90

Chapter 9   Your Emotions Carry Messages   102

PART 3: *Your Unbreakable Inner Compass*

Chapter 10   Guided by Your Gut   114

Chapter 11   Building Better Boundaries   124

Chapter 12   Bigger Than Your Body   135

Chapter 13   Who Are You? Like, Really...Who Are You?   147

Chapter 14   Staying Connected to Your Truth   **158**

Conclusion: Thriving, Not Striving   **168**

Acknowledgments   **172**

Additional Resources   **174**

References   **175**

Foreword

My friend broke her ankle last weekend. Successful, smart, and athletic, Jane is a woman in her sixties—"successful" by all cultural standards. She was distraught that she would have to be off her feet for the foreseeable future. But it wasn't missing her cherished daily hikes in nature, or time with her daughter who was her hiking companion, that most upset her. No, what agitated my friend about her broken ankle was simple... As she put it, "I'm going to get fat." In a culture that glorifies only one body type and pushes women to chase an ever-narrowing beauty standard, it's not enough to over-achieve; you have to over-achieve while also maintaining (or striving toward) a "fit" body, which we know is code for "thin."

Today, a thirty-five-year-old client reported that she'd signed up for another self-improvement seminar. Abby listens to podcasts on the way to and from work, gets up at 4 a.m. to go to the gym, and is always, proudly, "working" on herself. She allows herself no downtime—other than the precise amount she's been told is necessary—to get more done. She's drunk the cultural Kool-Aid: if she's productive enough, then *she's* enough. But when I ask Abby, "Do you feel like you're enough?" she answers without hesitation, "I can't even imagine what that would feel like." Despite all her productivity, she still doesn't believe she deserves to rest, let alone live by her own wants and needs. She believes any chance at "enough-ness" would be lost if she stopped striving, pushing, and denying herself—doing better. In truth, what the constant striving allows my client to feel is a little less *not enough*, as long as she keeps chasing the dream of perfection which she'll never attain and never have permission to attain.

Like my friend, my client, and the hundreds of emotionally exhausted, depleted women who've come through my door in the thirty years I've been a psychotherapist, I too grew up in the wellness and hustle cultures about which Paula writes so accurately, and heartbreakingly.

I grew up in an era when women were taught to be as small as possible—literally, to disappear; we learned to feel shame about our bodies unless they fit inside a tiny window of what was considered acceptable. I spent far too much of my life trying to outrun, starve, anesthetize, and avoid my body's experience and the feelings it carried. A triple "Type A," I drove myself hard to eradicate any sign that I might be "human" or be vulnerable in any way. The idea of having needs or limitations was off-the-table and shameful; there were and could be no cracks in the armor.

I'm now raising two daughters in this same toxic culture, watching as they, understandably, fall prey to the same challenges and obstacles we've all faced: the obsession with physical appearance and belief that their value is defined by how well they meet the standards our patriarchal culture sets for them. Despite all my understanding and encouragement, I watch them leaving *home*—their real home inside themselves—turning away from their truth, and relating to their bodies as objects to manage and control for the greater goal (and safety) of being likable. And I watch them suffer in the ways we all suffer as women chasing a destination to which we can never arrive.

I don't usually write forewords, but when Paula sent me the notes for her book, I knew, schedules be damned, that I wanted to lend my voice to this much-needed project. Paula's wisdom and guidance arise from her own lived experience of anxious perfectionism and body-image dissatisfaction, as well as her work with so many women, which is why her voice is filled with truth and compassion, and a ferocity she gathered, paradoxically, from being both a follower and escapee of the wellness and hustle cultures about which she writes.

In this book, the author teaches women to identify when we're chasing an unattainable, culturally assigned goal and ignoring our own authentic needs and values. She lays out a path for breaking free from the mental rules, self-criticism, and elaborate internal systems we construct to succeed and survive in our *"be beautiful, be productive, be perfect"* culture.

Most importantly, Paula refrains from telling the reader who to be, and instead helps her develop curiosity and compassion for her *own* experience. She encourages her to discover her inner world and what genuinely matters—to her. This is not another book that tells us how to be a more confident and productive version of ourselves, rather, it is about learning to trust our own wisdom, come home, and be who we actually are. In other words, *real* freedom.

—Nancy Colier, LCSW, Rev.,
    author of *The Emotionally Exhausted Woman*

Introduction: The Target Is Always Moving

I still remember the day I got my first B. It wasn't even a B; it was a B-*plus* on a history quiz. I was eleven years old, and I came home crying. Convinced it was a fluke, I begged my teacher to let me retake it. She relented, but apparently I just didn't know the American Revolution as well as I thought I did. On the second try, I got the exact same grade.

Suddenly, my little fifth-grader sense of self was in shambles. Who was I if I didn't get straight As? That was when I heard it—the voice in my brain. The one that chimed in anytime I made a mistake. It screamed at me, "You're supposed to be *smart!* You don't get Bs, you get As!" The only solution was to work harder. Maybe if I studied for twice as long, I could prevent this burning humiliation from ever happening again.

Throughout my life, I've had similar earth-shattering moments. I entered puberty and gained weight. My brain said, "*No! Stop!* You're supposed to be thin." Cue the dieting and disordered eating that ruled my life for the next few decades. I got rejected from my top-choice college. My brain said, "This wasn't the plan. You've ruined everything!"

You'd think that with so much emphasis on success, my brain would praise me when I finally reached my goals. But that was the most puzzling part. Anytime I achieved something, even something I worked really hard for, my brain would say "So what? Big deal!" I'd have the occasional flash of pride when I reached a goal, but it would subside as quickly as it arrived.

I could never quiet that voice pushing me to strive harder, achieve more. The voice kept promising me that I just needed to clear that next hurdle and I could finally land in a place where I would feel eternally worthy, happy, and confident. The promises were empty though. My achievements were never enough, never worthy of more than the tiniest moment of celebration. It became almost predictable, that inner voice quoting with dead seriousness Elle Woods's quip when she decides to go to Harvard Law School: "What, like it's hard?!"

The thing is, it *was* hard. It was *always* hard, and the target was always moving. It wasn't enough to excel at school or in my career; I was still failing if I didn't wake up early and hit the gym. It wasn't enough to pack homemade salads for lunch; I was still failing if I didn't also keep in touch with friends. I vacillated between eating as few calories as possible and bingeing on diet snacks. I flipped between studying obsessively and procrastinating. In every area of life, I believed I was falling short. I was a crappy friend, mediocre professional, lazy, and selfish. Worst of all, it was my own fault. I was the one who couldn't muster the discipline to stay on top of everything.

Somehow, other people didn't have these problems. In my everyday life and online, I compared myself to everyone around me and came up short. It was like I was absent on the day in elementary school when everyone learned the secret to success. Everyone else was able to get eight hours of sleep, wake up at the alarm, hit the gym, cook a healthy breakfast, crush their to-do lists, spend quality time with loved ones, drink enough water, keep their kitchens clean, rinse and repeat it all the next day. The wellness influencers could do it. My friends and family could do it. I was the only one falling short. The only reasonable conclusion was that *I* was the problem.

I spent my days consumed by the false belief that I could somehow achieve enough to quiet that inner critic. In graduate school, I came to understand that I was actually dealing with a cocktail of psychological conditions rooted in control-seeking behaviors. One of my professors used to say, "All research is *me*-search; we pursue the things that resonate most deeply with us." And so, it was no surprise that, when I became a psychologist, I developed a specialty in perfectionism, anxiety, and disordered eating.

At first glance, it may not seem like perfectionism and disordered eating come from the same place. But whether you're beating yourself up for slacking off during the workday or for a late-night pizza binge, the psychological mechanics are often similar. Both are rooted in a strong desire for self-control and the belief that self-control is an indicator of whether you deserve to experience satisfaction.

Many people who struggle with self-criticism and body image are also empathetic and highly sensitive. They instinctively accommodate everyone around them, often at their own expense. They are high achieving but incredibly hard on themselves, trapped in a never-ending game of whack-a-mole. Once one part of life feels like it's under control, their brains push them toward that next thing. They live with outside pressures telling them that they're the problem, and an inner critic echoing that sentiment.

I wrote this book for people who:

- feel intense pressure to keep up appearances, earn approval, or get things "right";

- never feel like they're doing enough to be proud of themselves;

- constantly think about what they "should" be doing when they try to rest or relax;

- attach their eating, body size, and physical appearance to how they feel about themselves as a whole;

- believe they lack self-control, discipline, or willpower (or flip between feeling super in control and going totally off-the-rails).

It is difficult to break free from these tendencies, especially when you live in a culture that celebrates discipline and self-punishment. The elusive hits of validation that come with "getting it right," however momentary, can become addictive. Unfortunately, they come at a high price: you devote your time, energy, and mental real estate to the chase. You never feel like you reach any destination to truly feel proud of, as life continues to present new challenges.

In Western culture, there is a great deal of emphasis on productivity. It can be hard to recognize when we're setting unrealistic standards because society reinforces a hustle mentality. There is also immense pressure to fit cultural standards of beauty. Thinness, fitness, and perfect health are held up as signs of achievement and, thus, signs of worthiness and acceptability. Entire industries are built on you believing that failure to achieve those standards is your own fault. They convince you that you just need to harness your attention, drink a shot of apple cider vinegar, and follow their ten-step program. So you keep striving for those goals, researching new fitness regimens, eating plans, and lifestyle changes to hack your way to "enough."

What if you could strip away the social conditioning that taught you to care about aesthetic beauty, productivity, and discipline, and determine whether you actually care about those things? You may protest at this suggestion, especially since society rewards people who conform to its ideals. But what if you could learn to tolerate the discomfort that comes with living outside the norm so you could also experience the freedom it brings?

It may feel scary or even impossible to imagine a life where you're not chasing unrealistic standards. However, when you stop chasing, you get the freedom to think for yourself, spend your time and money how you choose, and feel at home in your own mind and body, even when the outside world tries to make you reject yourself. After all, everyone has qualities that some will value and others will reject, and personality traits that serve as assets in some contexts and limitations in others. You weren't born believing yourself to be lazy or selfish. You were only *taught* to believe these things. It doesn't have to be this way. You can unlearn the things you've learned, and make space to actually enjoy your brief time on this planet.

The truth is that no matter how hard you work, you'll *never* be thin enough, successful enough, or worthy enough to rest. It's not because you're deficient; it's because you're chasing a moving target that is literally designed to keep you chasing. As long as you're turning to the outside world for instructions, you'll inevitably get stuck. Plus, regardless of whether or not you're matching up with those ideals, you'll never feel like "enough" because you cannot control what you feel inside.

In fact, efforts to control your cravings and fears typically backfire and end up controlling *you*. What you resist persists. The more you strive to feel worthy, the more controlled you are by the desire for worthiness. The more you focus on achieving your ideal body, the more finicky your body image becomes. The more you try to avoid eating sweets, the more anxious you feel when they're around. The more you cling to a plan, the more bothered you'll be when that plan gets derailed.

This book will teach you how to identify when you're wasting energy with toxic striving. It will help you figure out what you'd rather be spending that energy on—where your authentic priorities lie. Nobody knows you more intimately than you. Nobody else has been one-hundred percent privy to all of your thoughts and feelings. That means you have the most information on yourself. This book won't give you answers; it will help you discover your own answers.

You'll come away from this book with a sense of self-trust. You won't learn how to be more confident or productive; you'll learn how to be more *yourself*. You'll define your own version of a rewarding and meaningful life; listen to the guidance of your physical, mental, and emotional signals; and make decisions that align with what matters most to *you*.

To do this, we'll weave together research-backed tools from acceptance and commitment therapy (ACT) and intuitive eating (IE). Some tools will suggest that you write your answers in your journal (or if you prefer, in a notebook or on your phone); other tools can be downloaded at http://www .newharbinger.com/54063.

Both ACT and IE treat you as the expert on your own mind, body, and life. Instead of searching for the next diet or hack to tame your body or mind, you can live according to the qualities you most wish to embody. This book will guide you to:

- understand how and when you stopped trusting yourself and started living according to outside standards;

- uncover subconscious rules about what you eat and how you spend your time so you can evaluate whether those rules are helpful or harmful;

- set goals that align with your personal values instead of society's expectations;

- learn to take power away from restrictive and self-punishing thoughts so you can be kinder to yourself;

- understand your hunger, fullness, and cravings and use them to reclaim pleasure and satisfaction with food and beyond;

- learn how to be an observer of your emotions rather than letting them control you;

- stop criticizing your body and appearance, and view your body as more than a decorative object;

- set effective boundaries with anyone who makes you feel ashamed of yourself for how you look, how much you get done in your day, or anything else.

Even if this seems like a lot of work, I hope you'll stick with it. I assure you it will be far less exhausting than the toxic striving you've been doing. You don't have to be familiar with ACT or IE in order to start. You don't have to worry about learning clinical jargon or following a step-by-step recipe. The point of this book is to help you do the opposite: throw away the rulebooks and write your own life story. From now on, *you* are the expert on you.

A Job You Didn't Sign Up For

PART 1

CHAPTER 1

How You Were Brainwashed

When you were born, you were a ball of instincts. You cried when hungry. You cried when tired. You cried when frustrated. You didn't have very many ways of expressing yourself (crying was pretty much it), but you sure weren't shy about letting everyone around you know what you needed. When you were hungry, you didn't worry about how much you'd already eaten that day. When you were upset, you didn't feel self-conscious wailing in the middle of the grocery store. You were guided completely from the inside.

Somewhere along the way, you learned to silence those instincts. Perhaps an adult yelled at you for throwing a tantrum, so you learned that feeling upset was shameful. Maybe a doctor told your mom to be careful with your snacks, so some of your favorite foods became off limits. You started getting messages from every direction telling you what made you good, what made you bad, and what you needed to strive toward. Those messages seemed important; after all, they came from the people you loved and trusted most.

Along with instincts, every child is born with a temperament. Some babies are naturally fussy, others are more relaxed. Some babies constantly want to be held, others prefer to be left alone. Almost immediately, adults begin making value judgments about a child's nature, insinuating that some tendencies are more acceptable than others. Children learn whether they're funny, outgoing, brave, shy, smart, sweet, or stubborn. Some messages are given in terms of how they *shouldn't* be. "Don't cry! Don't eat too much. Don't be so sensitive." Other times, messages are framed as a comparison: "You're so much quieter than your brother!" These messages land in a child's psyche and begin to shape their perception of who they are and how they're supposed to be.

Messages like these are often well intentioned. Parents are tasked with raising children to become functional adults capable of contributing meaningfully to society. A large part of that task is teaching children to self-regulate so that by the time they're adults, they can manage their emotions without throwing a toddler-style temper tantrum. Unfortunately, lessons in self-regulation often get inadvertently twisted into lessons in self-silencing. This is particularly true for people socialized as female in a culture where females are rewarded for being agreeable and selfless. Chronically suppressing your needs and emotions, saying yes when you really wanted to say no, or being endlessly available to make sure others are comfortable can all be forms of self-silencing. These tendencies have been linked to higher rates of depression, eating disorders, chronic disease, and even premature death (Jakubowski et al. 2022; Maji and Dixit 2019; Ussher and Perz 2010).

It's impossible to move through life without outside influence, and often, outside influence is helpful. We have an instinct, follow that instinct, and then get feedback about whether the way we followed that instinct was effective. The problem is that many of us learn to listen *only* to external feedback, and completely ignore internal feedback. Eventually, we silence the voice inside of us telling us what we find meaningful and authentic. We learn that it's more important to satisfy the world around us than to satisfy ourselves.

To peek into how you might develop a habit of self-silencing, let's imagine that you're three years old. Your baby sister snatches your beloved doll right out of your hands. You're overwhelmed with anger. You cry and scream, but she doesn't give the doll back. You start hitting her in an attempt to cope with the intense rage filling your three-year-old body. Now you've got your mom's attention. She yells, "We do *not* hit!" Perhaps her intention was to communicate that the anger you're feeling is natural, but responding to it by hitting is not appropriate. However, instead of separating the emotion from the reaction, you learn that they are one and the same: *Anger is not okay.*

In another scenario, imagine your mom *does* acknowledge that anger is natural. She sees you hitting your sister and says, "I know you feel angry that she took your doll, but you're not allowed to hit." You learn what *not* to do when angry, but you don't learn alternatives. This leaves you confused;

what do you do next time anger arises? How do you regulate it effectively? Without further guidance, that confusion becomes shame, and shapes one of your strategies for getting through life successfully: *Avoid expressing anger.*

These experiences lay the foundation for our belief systems. While not set in stone, ideas of "how to be" set up camp in our unconscious minds from such a young age that we don't even recognize that they're beliefs. They simply seem like facts. What if, when you were that three-year-old child, your mom taught you to step outside when angry, take five slow deep breaths, and calm your body down? You might grow up learning how to validate your emotions, while still appropriately controlling your impulses. While there are many schools of thought on how to teach children to regulate, parents are often stretched thin. It is not always realistic that a parent will have the foresight, patience, and internal resources to coach their child through the scenario above. As a result, many children grow up feeling lost when strong emotions arise.

Parents and caregivers aren't our only sources on how to be. We're also conditioned by our surrounding culture. We're shaped by social systems telling us that some brains, bodies, and personalities are more desirable than others. In Western culture, ideals of productivity, discipline, self-control, and youthfulness prevail. Cultural critics have addressed these forces through many lenses: capitalism, white supremacy culture, grind culture, and productivity culture. This book will examine two facets of these social and economic systems as driving forces behind eating-, body-, and achievement-focused anxieties and obsessions: wellness culture and hustle culture.

Wellness Culture

In recent decades, there has been increasing cultural emphasis on health and, more nebulously, wellness. While it's human nature to seek pain relief, our obsession with wellness has spiraled beyond the basic desire for ease into an aspirational lifestyle that companies have been happy to pounce upon for financial gain. According to registered dietitian Christy Harrison (2023), the global wellness industry is valued at $4.4 trillion. We jump eagerly at whatever trend in health, fitness, medicine, and alternative medicine comes through the revolving door next. There is a glorification of "natural" remedies for ailments, eating "clean" and "whole" foods, and eschewing anything processed or containing additives or chemicals. At the same time, we want a quick fix, a pill or formula that provides guaranteed results. We're obsessed with *biohacking*, attempting to control health outcomes beyond what is realistic. We're allured by the promise of wellness influencers and alternative health providers who swear by their complicated nutritional formulas or miracle herbs and supplements.

While most people want to be well, the degree to which we pursue wellness may actually be making us sicker, if not physically, then certainly mentally. There is significant emotional consequence to obsessively controlling every aspect of one's well-being, from diet and exercise to pain management, blood sugar, and sleep. Sometimes, the fixation on health symptoms and preoccupation with finding answers can lead us down a rabbit hole of potentially dangerous, unregulated treatments or pursuing unnecessarily restrictive lifestyles. When you're convinced that a certain food, substance, or product is toxic, the anxiety you feel when around that product and the lengths you go to avoid it can be what's actually harming you, or at least exacerbating any real effects. Wellness culture preys on our existential anxiety "by promising to stave off death" (Harrison 2023).

The assumptions of wellness culture are inaccurate at best, and discriminatory and dangerous at worst. Wellness culture promotes *healthism*, the interweaving of goodness and morality with health. For many people, these healthist beliefs become religious; engaging in health practices makes you superior or virtuous, and *not* pursuing health makes you sinful. Healthism blames people for their health problems. This perspective is also ableist, denigrating people based on ability. Harrison (2023) refers to wellness as "the rich person's version of health," especially as social currency is awarded not just for being healthy, but for actively striving toward greater well-being, through seeing alternative health providers (often not covered by health insurance), buying special and costly organic cooking ingredients, and devoting time and resources to these pursuits that many individuals simply do not have.

One of the more prominent branches of wellness culture is diet culture. In *Anti-Diet: Reclaim Your Time, Money, Well-Being, and Happiness Through Intuitive Eating*, Christy Harrison (2019) describes diet culture as a system that "worships thinness and equates it to health and moral virtue...promotes weight loss as a means of attaining higher status...demonizes certain ways of eating while elevating others...[and] oppresses people who don't match up with its supposed picture of 'health,' which disproportionately harms women, femmes, trans folks, people in larger bodies, people of color, and people with disabilities, damaging both their physical and mental health."

While anyone can experience pressure to achieve unrealistic body ideals or attach morality to their health status, people socialized as female, people of color, sexual minorities, people in larger bodies, and people with disabilities often face the brunt of these pressures. The pressures themselves emanate from systems of patriarchy, racism, ageism, and ableism. Consider what's held up as the ideal body: it's often young, thin, white (or with Eurocentric features), abled, cisgender, and free of disease. In *Fearing the Black Body: The Racial Origins of Fat Phobia*, Dr. Sabrina Strings (2019) points out the intricate ways in which the glorification of thin bodies has sprung directly from racist beliefs. Diet culture and wellness culture work hand in hand with anti-Blackness, pathologizing the natural diversity across our species.

Cultural obsession with health and wellness has even led to the rise of a new type of eating disorder, *orthorexia nervosa*. Though not yet part of the *Diagnostic and Statistical Manual of Mental Disorders* (DSM, the manual used by healthcare professionals as a guide for mental health diagnoses), the diagnosis of orthorexia has been well-founded (López-Gil et al. 2023). Someone with orthorexia is preoccupied with eating in a way they deem healthy, which might mean eating "clean," avoiding processed foods, eating only organic, avoiding anything with additives, and so forth. While on the surface this might seem harmless, it can easily spiral into obsession and rigidity. Sadly, if someone engages in disordered eating and lives in a culture that praises those behaviors, their suffering can go unnoticed for a long time. Sometimes, even health professionals don't recognize an eating disorder until there are extreme consequences.

Diet culture tells us that body size is completely within your control. Wellness culture tells us that health is completely within your control. By diet culture's logic, it's your fault if you don't have the ideal physique. By wellness culture's logic, it's also your fault if you have health problems.

These assumptions are flat-out false. You cannot determine someone's health or habits by looking at them. Most of us know people who are naturally thin, despite eating nothing but fast food and sitting on the couch all day. On the flip side, there are plenty of people who are naturally larger, even if they run marathons and primarily eat nutritious foods. There are people who are thin with lots of health problems, and others who are fat with excellent health markers. Most of us know that health is complex. No matter how much spinach you eat, you can't control for genetics, early childhood environment, or the stress of discriminatory systems. Not everyone has access to quality health care or a safe environment in which to be physically active. These, and numerous other factors, affect our health.

It's important to remember that despite the false narrative pushed upon you that body size is a choice, bodies have *always* come in a variety of shapes and sizes. As Judith Matz and Ellen Frankel write in *Beyond a Shadow of a Diet* (2024), "Even if everybody ate the exact same foods and engaged in the same amount of daily activities, there would still be a wide variation of body sizes." For many, trying to fight a naturally larger body is like trying to make themselves taller or shorter. It just doesn't work long-term. Most people who lose any significant weight on purpose end up regaining most or all of it within two to five years (Bacon and Aphramor 2011; Mann et al. 2007). Since our culture isn't okay with weight regain, many people then embark on another attempt to lose weight…and eventually regain it once again. This pattern of losing, regaining, losing, and regaining weight is called *weight cycling.*

Weight cycling causes more harm to physical and mental health than remaining at a stable weight, even when that weight is higher. Research demonstrates that weight cycling increases risk of cardiovascular disease, heart attack, stroke, type 2 diabetes, cortisol production, binge eating, life dissatisfaction, and body image preoccupation (Bacon and Aphramor 2011; Brownell and Rodin 1994; Diaz, Mainous, and Everett 2005; Fothergill et al. 2016; Rhee 2017). In other words, trying to force your body to be smaller than it wants to be can lead to the same health problems you're trying to avoid by shrinking it!

Beyond the physical and mental health problems caused by weight cycling, this perspective perpetuates weight stigma. It's no surprise that weight stigma has toxic effects on health. It is stressful to experience judgment, bullying, and harassment in your daily life. That chronic stress can lead to high levels of cortisol, high blood pressure, heart disease, depression, isolation, anxiety, and avoidance of situations where one might experience shame. Research shows that experiencing weight stigma increases chances for developing an eating disorder. Thanks to weight stigma, health professionals frequently miss signs of eating disorders in larger patients, so larger patients may also have an increased chance of going without proper diagnosis or treatment for many more years than smaller patients (Haines et al. 2006; Neumark-Sztainer et al. 2002; Puhl 2019; Puhl and Brownell 2006). As you might imagine, living with an untreated eating disorder is also not great for health.

Whether or not you have experienced weight cycling or weight stigma, you have likely absorbed messages urging you to avoid weight gain. No matter your size, these messages can contribute to obsession with food or weight, body shame, and suffering. That's what consumed my client Tanya. When I got a voicemail from Tanya one Sunday morning, I could hear the desperation in her voice. She'd gone out the night before and, after several rounds of tequila shots, came home to lose herself in a binge-eating episode. In the span of an hour, she scarfed down a large pizza, a dozen chicken wings, and five donuts. She woke up with a nasty hangover, sharp stomach pains, and crushing guilt. She whispered, "What is *wrong* with me?! Will I *ever* be able to control myself around food?"

Tanya had struggled with food for her whole adult life. By age thirty-five, she had tried every detox and clean-eating plan out there, from Weight Watchers to macro counting to the Keto diet. She'd start determined. Sometimes she lost ten, twenty, or thirty pounds, and would feel a brief sense of accomplishment; then a happy hour or friend's wedding would throw off her game and she'd be back to late-night binges.

Tanya's secret nighttime eating was one of many things she beat herself up about. At work, with friends, and with her boyfriend, she felt she was always "too much"—too selfish, too impulsive, too loud, too sensitive. As the oldest daughter of Korean immigrants, Tanya spent her childhood walking a tightrope of specific beauty standards reinforced through the Korean and American media she followed. She felt an obligation to achieve financially and show her parents that their sacrifices had paid off. Despite her successful career as a nurse at a local children's hospital, she found her self-worth always came back to her appearance. She figured if she could just lose weight and actually keep it off, that would be enough to feel confident in other parts of her life. Things would finally fall into place.

Recognizing Wellness Culture Conditioning

Even if your story is different from Tanya's, you may resonate with her struggles. Many of us are taught that our success is not valid if we don't also lose weight or maintain a certain size. We learn to attach self-worth to our bodies and our perceived health. Take a moment to consider what you were taught about eating, size, and health. You may want to write your responses in a journal; you can also download the questions at http://www.newharbinger.com/54063.

As a child, who decided what you ate, when you ate, and how much you ate?

Growing up, did you think about food much? Did you ever have to worry where your next meal would come from?

Was food ever used for reward or punishment? If so, how?

Were certain types of foods ever limited or restricted? If so, what types?

Did you play sports or engage in physical activity as a kid? If so, did you enjoy that? Why or why not?

How were bodies discussed in your home? In your social environment (at school, with friends, or in your community)?

Was health emphasized in your home? How did the important people in your life define health, and what did they teach you about it?

Did you visit doctors or health professionals growing up? What messages did they give you about your health?

What TV shows, movies, magazines, books, and so on did you enjoy, and what did you learn from them about bodies and beauty?

Were you ever made to feel that your body was not acceptable? What was this like for you?

How do you feel about your body today?

How do your feelings about your body impact your relationship with food and/or physical activity?

This activity may bring up difficult memories or emotions. Go slowly if you need to. You may wish to process these questions with a trusted friend or therapist. As challenging as it may be to think about your past, understanding your conditioning is an important step toward unlearning messages that have hurt you.

Hustle Culture

Wellness culture isn't the only force that instills us with self-doubt. While wellness culture tells us to control our bodies and hack our way to optimal health, hustle culture says we should control our minds. Joe Ryle, director of the nonprofit 4 Day Week Campaign, explains hustle culture as the system whereby work dominates your time in "such an unnatural way that we have no time to live our lives." Productivity is treated as a priority above all else.

There is an overarching system of "hustle and grind," sometimes called hustle culture and sometimes called grind culture, nodding to the same concepts of pressure to overwork, emphasis on productivity over humanity, and glorification of self-sacrifice. In *Rest Is Resistance: A Manifesto*, Tricia Hersey (2022) describes grind culture as a "collaboration between white supremacy and capitalism." Hersey founded the Nap Ministry as a salve for racial trauma, a movement to reclaim rest and dreaming from the people and systems that commodified bodies, specifically Black bodies, and that continues to deprive people of their humanity. While the pressures for hustle and grind can affect anyone, the consequences of not complying are harshest for those who have historically been exploited for labor—in the United States, Black people, Indigenous people, and people of color who continue to face racism and systemic inequities.

For many who lived through the Great Recession of 2008, overworking has been both an economic necessity and familiar way of life. A GOBankingRates survey found that one in four Americans is working another gig or side job in addition to their full-time work. Perhaps to cope with the reality of a tough economic climate, social media and self-help circles popularized the idea that a "rise-and-grind" mentality would solve the struggle. Working long hours and taking on a side hustle became something to be admired (World Health Organization 2021; Huddleston 2019).

Working long hours isn't just bad for work-life balance; it's sometimes deadly. A 2021 analysis by the World Health Organization and the International Labour Organization found that between 2000 and 2016, the number of deaths from heart disease due to working long hours increased by 42 percent. The number of deaths from stroke due to working long hours increased by 19 percent. These health risks were prominent in people working fifty-five hours or more per week, compared to those who worked thirty-five to forty hours per week. This is without even accounting for the countless hours of invisible labor that many people put into household chores, childcare, and eldercare every day.

Like wellness culture, the premise of hustle culture is that you're completely in charge of your fate. If you're not totally crushing it at work, you're not hustling hard enough. Human beings aren't machines. We can't just put our nose to the grindstone and crank out work every waking moment until we die, yet we berate ourselves for not functioning this way. It's no wonder journalist Anne Helen Petersen (2020) nicknamed millennials "the burnout generation." Young adults, and increasingly, people of all ages, are suffering from the false belief that with hard work and discipline, it's possible to do everything.

That's what my client Allie discovered when we started exploring the things that were keeping her up at night. At twenty-nine, she had just been promoted to a management role at her company. On paper, she was living her best life. In reality, she felt constantly insecure. Her team saw her as a role model, but she couldn't imagine why anyone would aspire to be like her. Though she occasionally had moments where she felt like a successful manager, her mind would quickly remind her she was actually a lazy slob who couldn't muster the discipline to wake up early and exercise before work.

Allie figured if she was truly a boss, like the high-powered career women she saw on TV, she'd wake at five in the morning, go for a run, whip up a green smoothie before sliding into a size two pencil skirt and breezing into the office. She'd be learning a skill in her spare time and meditating before bed. Instead, she was watching the scale creep higher and ignoring the check engine light on her car. When she was on her game at work, she was slacking on her workouts. When she was making time to see friends, she was forgetting work deadlines. She was always guilty, always stressed, and constantly felt like she was disappointing somebody.

Recognizing Hustle Culture Conditioning

Allie's self-image relied heavily on her productivity. Even if your story differs from Allie's, you may relate to her self-criticism and feelings of inadequacy. As you did with wellness culture, you can uncover messages instilled in you from hustle culture. Feel free to focus on whichever questions resonate with you most. You can write your responses in your journal or download the questions at http://www.newharbinger.com/54063.

As a kid, what do you remember learning about success?

How did the adults in your life respond to your dreams and goals?

What qualities or characteristics did the adults in your life seem to respect or admire the most in each other?

What types of things did the adults in your life brag about or celebrate? What milestones or achievements were they most proud of?

What kinds of things did the adults in your life act ashamed of or gossip about?

How was relaxation or rest treated in your family? Did you ever see the adults in your life taking breaks or simply doing nothing? Were you allowed to take breaks or relax if there was still work to be done?

These days, what do you most criticize yourself about?

When are you proudest of yourself?

What do other people criticize about you?

Wellness and hustle cultures tell us that our value lies in external measures of success—how much money we make, how physically fit our bodies look, how early we wake up. There is a "right" way to be, and that way involves crushing your goals while looking effortlessly hot. Discipline and willpower are presented as social currency, tickets to a good life full of health, wealth, and happiness.

For those who struggle with perfectionism and control, productivity and body image are two sides of the same coin. Though they seem like separate issues, both stem from a culture that glorifies the grind. If you relate to Tanya, you may notice that even if your internal rules are mostly about eating and weight, there's a piece of the formula related to overall success. If you relate more to Allie, you may notice that even if most of your rules are about being productive, there's still a piece of the formula that involves looking the part.

WELLNESS CULTURE		HUSTLE CULTURE
To eat right, exercise, and make "healthy choices"	You need *discipline*	To "do the work" and hack your productivity
To resist temptation	You need *willpower*	To resist distraction
Give in to temptation	You're weak if you...	Take breaks or relax
Attaining the "ideal" body and optimal health	Hard work will result in...	Crushing your goals and achieving success

For better or worse, conditioning is a fact of life. But sometimes the things you were conditioned to strive toward become all-consuming. You become a target chaser, addicted to the praise and validation you get for hitting the mark on externally imposed goals. Deep down, you feel empty because you're not chasing what matters to *you*.

Once you can see that these values come from wellness and hustle culture, you get to decide whether they are the most important things to you. While it's understandable to want the praise and privilege afforded to those who strive, the chase is never-ending. Even if society continues to glorify the chase, you have permission to reject societal ideals that don't resonate for you. After all, you're the only one living *your* life!

Reevaluating Your Conditioning

You've likely been taught some things that have helped you and others that have not. This exercise can help you uncover those lessons and organize them in terms of what you'd like to keep, revise, and let go.

Part 1: Identifying Your Conditioned Values

In your journal, reflect on these questions:

When you were growing up, what made your parents or caregivers proud?

What were you praised for? Were your siblings praised for the same things or different things? What about your peers?

What made your parents or caregivers upset, angry, or disappointed? What did you get punished or get into trouble for? (If you didn't get into trouble, what types of things did you know not to do so that you could avoid trouble?)

What daily habits or routines were part of your family? (For example, hygiene, eating, exercise, work, relaxation, socializing)

What emotions were frequently expressed in your household when you were growing up?

Were all emotions allowed, or were some feelings more acceptable while others needed to be hidden or ignored?

Were some members of the household allowed to express certain emotions that others weren't?

What was this like for you?

Part 2: Keeping What Works, Rethinking the Rest

Read over your responses. What themes do you notice? For example, if you were praised for being sweet and well-behaved, perhaps you learned: "It's good to follow rules and not make waves." You may have learned to value orderliness or obedience. If your parents got upset when you didn't share toys, you may have learned to value generosity.

In your journal, list two or three themes in the lessons you were taught growing up:

What did you learn was important in life?

What did you learn about how you were supposed to look?

What about how you were supposed to behave?

What personality traits did you learn you should try to embody?

Considering these themes, is it worth holding on to any of the values or lessons you were instilled with? Which ones? Which values or lessons might be worth rethinking?

In chapter 2, you'll work on strengthening the beliefs you want to keep and letting go of the ones that aren't helping you live your best life.

CHAPTER 2

You Were Never
the Problem

I went to middle school with a girl named Becca who exuded genuinely chill vibes. Like many twelve-year-old girls at the turn of the millennium, she had braces, acne, and a Trapper Keeper covered in Lisa Frank stickers. But unlike the rest of us, who were either clinging to a place in the popular group (not me) or desperately seeking approval from said popular group (definitely me), Becca did her own thing. When the rest of the girls started bringing salads and fat-free pudding cups for lunch, Becca ate the sandwiches and chips she liked. When the other kids started wearing double-layered polo shirts, Becca stuck to her floral-print tank tops.

Nothing seemed to faze Becca. If she got a question wrong in front of the class, she just shrugged and said, "Oops!" If I got a question wrong, I'd refuse to raise my hand for the rest of the year. Once her Capri Sun exploded, and she spent the afternoon covered in red juice stains. I was vicariously mortified, but Becca found it hilarious. Becca's attitude was so foreign to me that it seemed like it must be a façade. But the more I got to know her, the more I understood that she was just a secure person.

While I never asked, I'm sure there were moments when Becca felt self-conscious or embarrassed. No human is completely immune from these feelings. However, she had an easygoing personality and didn't focus on others' opinions. Despite living in the same culture of toxic striving, Becca was able to ignore pressures and simply live her life. In hindsight, I was probably baffled by her outlook because she represented a value I so badly wanted to embody. I wanted to be comfortable being my authentic self, but I was miles away from understanding what that even meant.

As we explored in chapter 1, we're each born with a temperament that colors how we interpret the world. Being naturally even-keeled and unflappable can help insulate someone against cultural pressures. In much of her work, writer and activist Ragen Chastain mentions *personality privilege*, or the concept that possessing certain personality traits makes it easier to move through society. Openness, boldness, and extraversion can make it easier to socially network or advocate for yourself when you need something. Those who are naturally introverted or anxious can face more barriers in these same scenarios.

On top of nature variables, we are all affected by nurture variables. Your environment can both harm you and help you. Conditioning happens at many levels, from your own family unit all the way up to your country or region of the world. Protective factors are usually issued at the innermost levels: family, social circles, and community. Even if the larger society operates with assumptions of wellness and hustle cultures, if you're in a subculture or family that values different priorities, you might easily brush off wellness and hustle messages as untrue and unimportant.

Many identity factors can also provide someone with unearned social privilege, protecting them from pressures to hide or change themselves. In Western cultures, being white, male, cisgender, thin, straight, abled, upper class, and healthy can shield someone from the toxic messages of wellness and hustle cultures. Conversely, if you don't fit that mold, you might internalize the message that the standards are different for you. Instead of growing up with constant reminders of what you're capable of achieving, you grow up being told to change, hide, or downplay aspects of yourself simply to survive. As we explored in chapter 1, everyone can experience pressure to strive for the narrow, rigid standards of wellness and hustle cultures, but that pressure is harshest on people who are further from what the culture holds up as worthy. Of course, fitting cultural standards of acceptability does not prevent stress or hardship, but it does minimize stress and hardship that comes from experiencing discrimination and other systemic injustice.

None of us can truly understand what it's like to move through the world in a body or identity other than our own. However, we can open our minds and hearts to better respect differences—in ourselves and in others. We can challenge assumptions about what makes a person successful, who we consider attractive, and who we aspire to be like. We can change the way we engage with cultural norms and seek opportunities to celebrate and embrace the rich diversity of our species. Social privilege is not a choice, nor do we choose the type of environment we're born or raised in.

However, we are far from passive beings simply existing as life happens to us. Humans have the unique capacity for critical thinking, and we can use this ability to shift how we engage with both our inner and outer worlds. As you start unbraiding the rope of your own unique nature and nurture variables, you can recognize how your personality traits, identity factors, and social conditioning influence your worldview. Becoming aware of these variables can empower you to stop striving for things you don't align with.

I spent a long time trying to be more even-keeled, easygoing, extraverted...basically trying to be less *me*. It never occurred to me that my neuroticism, sensitivity, and conscientiousness could serve as strengths. Sure, people who are naturally more conscientious may struggle needlessly. That's half the premise of this book. Yet these same characteristics can also make someone organized, caring, ambitious, motivated, generous, and reliable. Any quality can be an asset in some situations and a limitation in others. Someone super laid-back with an attitude of "It'll be fine!" might be at risk of minimizing the seriousness of a crisis. Meanwhile, someone more conscientious or attentive to details might be quick to recognize that same problem and spring into action.

Of course, none of us is a one-dimensional archetype. Even the most neurotic among us can cultivate a sense of calm, and even the most outgoing person might get shy in a group of strangers. Plus, no personality trait is inherently good or bad. You're not better or worse than anyone else for being introverted, boisterous, or skeptical. In fact, that diversity of personalities is key for our species to thrive. I'm more of a worrier, while my husband is more easygoing. In his words, he's the gas and I'm the brakes—and we need both! If we were both like him, we might overlook tedious but important errands. If we were both like me, we certainly wouldn't have as much fun. That personality difference allows for a healthy partnership. Nothing is wrong with being whatever way *you* naturally are. By respecting your nature, you can learn to work *with* your inner world, not against it.

In graduate school, my friend and fellow anxious striver conducted her dissertation study on perfectionism (further proof that all research is "me-search"). It turns out that not all perfectionism is soul sucking. The variety I knew best, of relentless self-criticism, rigid thinking, and obsessive pursuit of unrealistic standards, was actually what the research termed maladaptive perfectionism (Lo and Abbott 2013). On the other hand, adaptive perfectionism involves striving with excitement and curiosity. Unlike maladaptive perfectionism, which deems you a failure if you don't reach your goals, adaptive perfectionism is about striving for excellence *without* attaching your self-worth to whether you achieve it. Instead of trying to get rid of perfectionist tendencies, those of us who are natural strivers can harness that quality as a strength.

For example, when I get really invested in a piece of writing, I can spend several days, weeks, even months retooling it. I will write and rewrite the same few paragraphs, tinkering with syntax until I'm satisfied. When I'm walking my dog or watching TV, I find myself noodling on that section. When I'm operating with adaptive perfectionism, I liken my writing process to that of a sculptor. I thrive in the process of striving. It excites me, rather than stressing me out. I enjoy the work of shaping and reshaping the same lump of clay until it feels ready to throw in the kiln.

This certainly doesn't mean my writing process is always harmonious. I still contend with a harsh inner voice telling me nothing I do is ever good enough. Yet when I can accept (and on a good day, embrace) my perfectionistic tendencies, I discover a quirky beauty in being this way. There is no right or wrong way to be. We don't all need to be chill and unbothered. If you're more of a striver, you can harness that inclination to strive, and use it to strive toward what you authentically care about.

Time, Money, and Mental Real Estate

To say Allie was a little compulsive about her slide decks would be an understatement. The night before her presentations to the senior staff at her company, she'd stay late at the office meticulously selecting fonts and transitions. Part of her felt silly, but another, louder part was sure she needed to double- and triple-check everything if she hoped to be taken seriously. She agonized over every decision, from choosing her outfit to choosing a health insurance plan.

One afternoon shortly after she was promoted, Allie watched a male colleague present a sales pitch. His slides were simple—black text on a white background. His outfit was equally simple—comfortable loafers and a T-shirt. Allie was instantly judgmental. What kind of underachiever thought he could present like that and be taken seriously? Except, she realized, he *was* being taken seriously. Nobody seemed to care about his slide design, or his outfit, for that matter. They were more focused on his ideas.

Allie wondered what it would be like to take a page from his book. She imagined presenting to her team without the distraction of high heels pinching her feet, but it seemed wrong. Everything she was conditioned to believe told her the standards were different for someone like her. While a white male colleague could rely on his intellect alone, Allie needed to not only have great ideas but also package and present them flawlessly.

Still, a seed was planted that afternoon. She wondered what would happen if she loosened up and wasn't so concerned with looking polished. What would it be like to throw on a sweater, go to work and just do her job? When would she stop feeling like an impostor who was one missed email away from being fired? Allie brought these reflections to her next therapy session. She began to explore what it was costing her to seek these standards.

Allie's focus on being organized and polished was not random; it was the result of lifelong social messaging. Allie was a larger-bodied Cuban woman. She had few examples of people who looked like her in high-powered corporate positions, but the ones she saw dressed impeccably and never missed a beat. She internalized a set of standards that seemed vital for success, and she developed extensive rituals to help her achieve them.

Once Allie brought her beliefs about appearance and success from her unconscious mind out to consciousness, she could recognize what they'd cost her. She was able to ask herself whether it was worthwhile to keep striving for these standards. That's what the next exercise is designed to help you do—uncover standards you've been unwittingly chasing, and figure out whether it's worthwhile to continue striving for them.

The Cost of Compliance

Using your journal or downloading this exercise at http://www.newharbin ger.com/54063, write down a belief about what you're supposed to look like or accomplish.

Pick something that has made you feel inadequate or self-conscious. Remember, a belief that seems trivial to one person can be a source of shame for someone else. When I completed this exercise, one belief I identi-fied was "*I am supposed to have clear, smooth skin.*" I picked this because it's caused me plenty of stress over the years, while for someone who has a naturally clear complexion, that belief probably wouldn't trigger as much emotion.

If you're having trouble identifying a belief to use, try completing these sentences with whatever pops into your head:

My body is supposed to have/be/look more…

My body is supposed to have/be/look less…

My skin should be…

My hair should be…

I'm lazy if I…

I'm selfish if I…

I'm a bad friend if I…

I'm a bad partner if I…

I'm a bad son/daughter/sibling/parent if I…

At work I should be…

I hate that I'm so…

I should be more…

You can add other beliefs to this list for completion.

Next, list as many ways as you can remember that you've tried to comply with this belief throughout your life.

Were any of these strategies effective at helping you comply with your belief? Consider whether any strategies helped permanently, temporarily, or partially, or didn't make a difference.

What have these efforts cost you in terms of time, energy, and money? Some questions to consider here:

How much time have you spent thinking about the "problem" or exploring solutions?

How much money have you spent on tools, products, or services to address the belief?

How much energy have you dedicated to this topic, and what has it taken you away from: sleep, social time, time with family or loved ones, activities and hobbies, vacations? (You don't have to know exact amounts. Just make an educated guess.)

How have your attempts to comply with the belief impacted your physical and emotional well-being?

Have you ever been successful at achieving the standard? If so, how did that success affect you physically, mentally, and emotionally?

How have you felt about yourself when you tried and failed to achieve the standard?

What would be different if you no longer felt pressure (from yourself or anyone else) to strive for this standard?

You can repeat this exercise with any other belief that's been a source of self-consciousness. The goal is to take stock of the resources you've devoted to "solving" the area(s) you've felt deficient in.

You're the only one who can know whether your investment is worthwhile. Maybe when you do this activity, you'll discover that some of your strategies are working, while others are draining you and taking you away from things that matter to you.

For me, the quest for clear skin has had an abysmal return on investment. Maybe if the first thing I tried had worked well, my glowy face and I would have just skipped off into the sunset to live happily ever after. Instead,

I sunk years of resources and energy into a pursuit that only ever worked temporarily before my skin would inevitably break out again. I spent countless hours in dermatologist offices, pharmacy lines, and internet rabbit holes. I tried powerful prescription drugs with horrific side effects. I spent God knows how much money on special facials. I poured mental energy into hiding scars and blemishes. I frequently felt self-conscious and ashamed.

When I stopped to reflect, the endeavor felt superficial and distracting. The energy I put toward pursuing beauty was at odds with my personal values. I felt icky upholding the idea that any human's worth (including my own) was based on attainment of some impossibly narrow aesthetic. I resented putting so much time and money into something I was conditioned to care about, when there were so many other, more meaningful aspects to my life. I'll admit that these days I'm not *not* doing any crazy skin stuff, but I'm much less invested in it. If I start getting fixated, I redirect my energy toward things I actually care about. The more I focus on my relationships, passions, and interests, the less important my skin feels.

You don't have to completely overhaul your habits and routines in order to start rejecting harmful beliefs. This stuff is complicated. You're contending with a lifetime of conditioning, plus continued exposure to messages telling you to keep striving. It's understandable if part of you wants to stop, but another part of you still clings to the striving strategies. The key is to think about how it affects your quality of life.

Depending on what you're struggling with and the extent of stigma or pressure you face, some practices will feel much riskier than others to challenge. Although my skin has caused me shame, strangers don't harass me about it on the street. My acne doesn't prevent me from accessing necessary health care or subject me to abuse, the way someone might experience if, for example, they are in a larger body and decide to stop trying to lose weight, or if they are openly trans, nonbinary, or gender nonconforming in an environment that promotes traditional expressions of gender. No matter who you are, you shouldn't have to punish yourself for deviating from oppressive standards. You're not the problem, even if society has led you to believe you are. The problem is, and always has been, the narrow standards you've been told to attain.

The standards and expectations upheld by the dominant culture may not disappear anytime soon. However, you get to decide whether you buy into those expectations. When any of us change how we engage with the world around us, there is a ripple effect. As we reach a critical mass, the standards themselves begin to change.

Getting honest about this stuff isn't easy. If you value inclusivity, you might feel ashamed to realize you've been striving for standards rooted in racism, misogyny, ableism, and ageism. You might feel angry, resentful, or sad to consider what these efforts have cost you. As dietitian Christy Harrison (2019) so aptly points out, diet culture (and, we could add, wellness and hustle) can be a "life thief," stealing your time, money, energy, and well-being while plying you with false promises of health, status, and happiness.

If you've ever taken a Psych 101 class, you're probably familiar with the term *cognitive dissonance*. This happens when we get information that contradicts our existing beliefs and wow, is it uncomfortable! It's like learning that Santa Claus is really your mom putting out presents and eating the cookies. Part of you wants to cling to the original belief—"He's real, darn it!"—while another part of you grapples with the hard truth.

Sometimes it seems easier to keep buying into the original belief. After all, you've gotten this far in life playing by the rules of the dominant culture, so why not continue? To be clear, this *is* an option. However, this strategy may not work long-term. A seed of doubt has been planted, so it may get harder and harder to stay in denial. Luckily, you also have other, more compassionate options.

In their body image research (2020), Drs. Lexie and Lindsay Kite examined how people responded to situations that affected their perception of their bodies, like being bullied, sexually assaulted, gaining or losing weight, or having a baby. They called these experiences *disruptions* because they have the potential to disrupt someone's relationship to their body. They discovered that following a disruption, people engage in one of three coping strategies. They either:

sink deeper into shame, turning to things that harm, punish, or numb them from their bodies, like disordered eating, drugs, alcohol, or self-harm;

hide or fix the things they deem unacceptable, through strategies like cosmetic surgery, makeup, baggy clothes, or avoiding situations where they don't want to be seen (for example, declining invites to the beach to avoid being seen in a swimsuit);

rise with resilience, which involves coming to terms with their feelings and experience, and letting the challenging situation make them stronger.

The Kites's research demonstrated that people who rise with resilience have more peaceful relationships with their bodies and derive self-worth from who they are, not what they look like. Although this model focuses on body image, you may find it useful for things you feel insecure about beyond your looks. When you fall behind on emails, instead of berating yourself (sinking deeper into shame) or staying up all night to catch up (attempting to fix), you can offer yourself compassion. You might say to yourself, *I'm not a productivity machine. Everyone falls behind sometimes. Which emails are priorities right now, and what can wait?*

If you asked someone at the end of their life to identify experiences that added richness and value to their time on this planet, you'd get a variety of answers. You might hear about reaching milestones, overcoming challenges, or developing meaningful relationships. It's possible that some will mention six-pack abs, thigh gaps, or seven-figure bank accounts. However, for many people, those aren't the standout experiences that bring lasting meaning or purpose. Often, we get caught up chasing superficial metrics because we've been conditioned to chase them, not because we value them deep down.

Psychologist Abraham Maslow (1943) popularized the concept of *self-actualization* as the ultimate goal that healthy, stable humans will strive toward. Assuming a person has met their most basic needs (food, water, shelter) and is physically, mentally, and emotionally comfortable, they will seek opportunities to live out passions and fulfill their potential. In other words, self-actualization is our species' most advanced pursuit. At our best, we're not striving with desperation, seeking to fill a void or compensate for what we believe we lack. When we come from a place that is secure and authentic, striving is a unique way that humans grow and evolve.

Striving looks different for each person. Although the dominant culture promotes a certain type of striving, that may not be the most meaningful pursuit for you. There's a reason why my pursuit of clear skin seems important yet leaves me feeling empty and ashamed. Meanwhile, my desire to continue growing as a psychologist, friend, and partner feels deeper and less dependent on outside validation. One of those pursuits comes from rules and messages I've absorbed, while the other is more innate.

The dominant culture glorifies certain characteristics and values over others, but you do not have to automatically accept those things as important. Because cultural conditioning can be so powerful, the values instilled in us may often feel like rules, rather than options. It can feel risky to reject them, as if you're breaking rules, but the rules are fake. If the things that wellness and hustle cultures tell you to care about aren't truly important or fulfilling to you, then you don't have to keep chasing them.

You can't completely eliminate negative self-talk; everyone has these thoughts sometimes. You also can't completely avoid harmful messaging from the outside world, so you may always face some degree of pressure. However, you can cultivate a more compassionate, flexible, and balanced inner world to help you stay resilient when negative thoughts arise and when external pressures creep in. The next chapter will help you uncover the rules you've internalized about how you should look, act, and spend your time. You'll explore how your own thoughts and self-talk uphold those rules, and learn strategies for shifting your inner dialogue.

CHAPTER 3

How You Learned the Rules

Tanya sat in the breakroom at work trying to estimate how many pretzels she'd just eaten. Earlier that month, she'd started using a calorie-tracking app to keep herself accountable. If she finished the day within her calorie limit, that day's square on the calendar filled in green. If she went over, it filled in red. If she had more than one red day this week, she would cancel her weekend brunch plans. The bully in her brain would criticize her until she came up with a plan to compensate.

That evening, she came home and ate the same dinner she'd had all week: chicken, steamed broccoli, and a cup of brown rice. She brushed her teeth to curb temptation to eat dessert, marked the day as complete in her app, and was relieved as another square filled in green. Before bed, she filled three bubbles on her habit tracker: "Bed by 9:30" *check*, "Work out" *check*, "Meal prep for tomorrow" *check*. Today was a good day. Maybe if she did a little extra cardio, she would even let herself splurge on a few mimosas this weekend.

Discipline was modeled for Tanya from a young age. She remembered her parents waking up at five in the morning, her father catching the early train to work and her mother packing homemade lunches for her and her sister before heading to twelve-hour nursing shifts. She knew her role, too. She was supposed to make her bed every morning and do her homework as soon as she arrived home each afternoon. As a child, she listened dutifully to her parents. As an adult, she listened dutifully to the wellness gurus she followed on social media.

Nobody sat her down and told her when to go to bed or what constituted an appropriate dinner, yet she came to understand there was a set of "correct" habits. These rules would lead to success and well-being. When she followed them, the bully in her mind sometimes let her rest. She would feel happy and confident, like she'd cracked the code. When she messed up, the bully got cruel and insulting. She'd spiral into shame.

Like Tanya, each of us has a set of internal rules governing what we are supposed to do. Not everyone's rules are the same; they depend on what you were instilled with and what messages you're surrounded by. Some rules might be helpful; they can provide a moral framework or guidance on how to maintain harmony. However, for people predisposed to toxic striving, the internal rulebook gets thicker and thicker as you absorb messages from wellness and hustle cultures on how to optimize your routines to do things "right." You may have rules for what to do with a free hour, what to choose from the menu at dinner, what your home should look like, how you should parent, how to dress, when to go to bed and wake up, and what to post on social media, pressuring you to perform at the highest level at every moment.

While wellness culture instills rules about eating, exercise, and health practices, hustle culture instills rules about focus and productivity. These rules are often so ingrained that you may not be conscious of them. They pop up in the form of all-or-nothing thought patterns that convince you there is a right and wrong choice for what to do and how to be in every situation. The inner rules might lead you to dismiss or overanalyze internal cues for hunger, tiredness, desires, and cravings. You may think you're "good" for denying yourself pleasure or pushing yourself to ignore discomfort.

In *Never Enough: When Achievement Culture Becomes Toxic—and What We Can Do About It*, journalist Jennifer Wallace (2023) explores how children in high-achieving communities absorb the message that their worth is directly tied to their accomplishments. Through pressure to fill their schedules with advanced placement classes, competitive sports, and extracurricular activities, kids learn that they matter only if they're achieving. Not only is it important to optimize productivity and performance to get into a "good" college, get a "good" job, and have a "good" life, it's also a reflection on whether you matter to the people you love. While this mentality is fostered in privileged communities where people have the resources to fixate on achievement, these are often the people with high social influence, shaping a striving-focused culture. It's no wonder so many people become obsessed with excellence and terrified of mediocrity.

While everyone's optimization rules are a bit different, they involve certain hallmarks: all-or-nothing thinking, emphasis on discipline, and moral judgment. Your rules might push you to exercise even when tired, compulsively check work emails from bed, or deny yourself something pleasurable like a vacation or a brownie. They might give you extreme guilt anytime you do something you've been taught to view as selfish or irresponsible. The rules can shape-shift, but they'll always make you feel like you're not good enough.

In the intuitive eating framework, rules about what, when, and how much to eat are referred to as the *diet mentality*. Even if someone doesn't follow a specific diet, they still may have ideas about the "correct" way to eat, both to lose weight (or avoid gaining weight) and to be healthy. While diet mentality refers to rules about food, you can think of this concept as part of an overarching set of optimization rules that you carry around internally, encompassing all beliefs about food, physical activity, health practices, and productivity. You may be so deeply entrenched in these rules that you lose connection with your cues. You may rarely, if ever, ask yourself what would be satisfying. When you crave something that goes against the rules, whether a cupcake or some alone time, you may feel frustrated with yourself for wanting something you shouldn't have.

Optimization rules can even consume your nonwaking hours. In the last few decades, sleep management has become a mainstay for strivers. A 2023 report from Emergen Research noted that in 2022, the global sleep economy and sleep aid market was worth about $512.8 billion. Sleep-tracking gadgets are designed to show how much "quality" sleep you're getting. Melatonin supplements, noise machines, weighted blankets, eye-shades, and wearable devices promise to optimize sleep, ostensibly so you'll awake early and refreshed, ready to crush more goals. I even had a client so preoccupied with his sleep metrics that he would lay in bed ruminating about whether he'd get high-quality sleep. He was being kept awake by the pressure he felt to get a good night's sleep!

Optimization rules don't account for the natural differences from one person to the next, and one moment to the next. Just as human bodies are naturally diverse, so are emotional and cognitive landscapes. Attention and energy ebb, flow, and vary day to day. Not everyone is wired to work best between the hours of 9:00 a.m. and 5:00 p.m. Not everyone thrives when meetings and lunch breaks are scheduled by someone else. Some people are morning larks and others are night owls. Some focus best in a noisy coffee shop while others need silence. You may have developed optimization rules as a way to control your productivity and output, but those rules don't account for your natural inclinations or fluctuating needs on a given day.

As psychologists will tell you, all behavior has a purpose. Attempts to follow optimization rules may actually be attempts to protect yourself or seek control over your well-being. For example, you might have rules about eating and exercise that are supposed to protect you from gaining weight (and experiencing weight stigma). What happens when your rules fail you, and you gain weight because your body drives you to binge eat after an unsustainable period of restriction (a phenomenon we'll discuss in chapter 6)? What happens when your body simply gets bigger because bodies change as they go through puberty, childbirth, or natural aging processes?

Rules about wellness come from efforts to protect you from illness and disease. What happens when you hydrate, take supplements, get quality sleep, and *still* get sick? Most people develop health problems through no fault of their own. Health is multifaceted, and outcomes can be related to aging, genetics, stress, and much more. Similarly, rules about excelling at work are supposed to protect you from getting fired. What happens when you work yourself into the ground and still lose your job? Optimization rules promise full control if you follow them perfectly, but even following them perfectly won't protect you from hardship. Your health, well-being, and success can't be hacked because you're a living, breathing organism.

On the surface, optimization rules seem like they're helping you stay on track but actually, they just make you feel inadequate. Rules can give you a steady supply of hypercritical ammunition to shoot at yourself, in the form of automatic thoughts. Did you know that on any given day, you have more than six thousand thoughts zipping through your mind (Tseng and Poppenk 2020)? You probably aren't aware of all of them. Instead, it can seem like thoughts are coming from an all-knowing narrator, an inner guru if you will.

Spotting Your Thoughts

Your thoughts aren't *actually* narrating your daily life; they're just plain ol' words in your brain. In fact, much of those six thousand thoughts are utter nonsense. We all have random, unhelpful thoughts on a regular basis. Yet the ones that bother us are the ones that stick around the longest and feel true. Often, these are optimization-based thoughts, the ones pushing you to keep chasing that moving target of "good enough." To throw the metaphorical rulebook into the garbage, first recognize the rules that are most prominent in your life and swap them out for more compassionate messages.

Part 1: Automatic Thought Log

One way to uncover optimization rules is to start a thought log. At regular intervals throughout the day, pause and pay attention to your automatic thoughts. Try setting an alarm to go off once an hour for a few days. When the alarm sounds, pause and notice what your mind was just telling you. Start a note in your journal to log the thoughts. Write down what was happening and what you were doing when the thought popped up.

You can also log thoughts outside of those "alarm bell" moments. For instance, you might notice thoughts chiming in at certain junctures, like when you start to feel hungry, when you look in the mirror, when you start a project, or when you notice an incomplete task, like a pile of unfolded laundry or dishes.

Remember, the goal is to simply begin noticing automatic thoughts; you don't need to try to change anything. Once you've gotten the hang of noticing thoughts without judgment, you're ready to move on to the next part of this activity, which will help you identify the nature of your automatic thoughts.

Part 2: Rules-Based or Compassionate?

Below are several statements someone's brain might say to them on a typical day. Using what you've learned about mental optimization rules, try to determine the flavor of each statement as either rules based or compassionate. You can write an R beside those that strike you as based on optimization rules, and C by the ones that land as compassionate.

_____ 1. "I ate so badly today. I never should have ordered that pizza."

_____ 2. "I'd like to get to the office early tomorrow to prepare for my meeting. I think the extra time will help me go in calmer."

_____ 3. "I barely drank any water today. I'll go fill my bottle now so that I don't get a headache."

_____ 4. "I should have remembered to call my friend on her birthday; I'm such a bad friend."

_____ 5. "I'm being too sensitive about not getting that promotion. It really isn't a big deal; other people have much worse problems."

_____ 6. "I could use some downtime tonight. I think I'll leave the laundry until tomorrow."

_____ 7. "I need to work out, I've been a lazy slob all week."

_____ 8. "I shouldn't be watching TV right now; I should be meditating."

_____ 9. "I need to eat vegetables and take my supplements every day or else I'll get sick."

_____ 10. "I thought I'd be finished by now but this project is taking longer than I expected. I still want to get home for dinner with my family. I think I'll ask my boss for an extension."

Was it difficult to discern between rules-based and compassionate messaging? Remember, what makes a message compassionate is the delivery style. A rules-based message will push you to ignore instincts, needs, or desires and punish you for anything less than perfect. A compassionate message encourages you to do something that aligns with your values, honors your needs, or helps you learn from a mistake. Optimization rules tie your performance and productivity to your worth, while compassionate messages account for the nuances of being a whole human being.

Answers: 1) R; 2) C; 3) C; 4) R; 5) R; 6) C; 7) R; 8) R; 9) R; 10) C.

Red Flags of a Rule

Here are some red flags that you're dealing with a rule:

It's phrased as a demand. Rules often contain command language—words like "should," "need to," "can't" or "must." While not all rules are harmful (for example, "I should refrain from violence" tends to be a useful rule for living in a peaceful society), optimization rules can be rigid and disregard natural ebbs and flows to our energy levels and needs.

It encourages rigidity. Rules often contain words like "never" or "always," but even helpful rules can have exceptions. Following a rule of "I should always refrain from violence" may be useful in 99.9 percent of situations, but harmful in the rare situation where you need to defend yourself from an attacker.

It links your performance to your worthiness. Rules imply that you're bad, wrong, or deficient in some way if you don't achieve a particular standard. They can make you feel undeserving of love or anything good in life when you can't meet an impossible standard.

It reeks of judgment. Rules put you (or others) into categories of inferior versus superior based on arbitrary metrics (how much one eats, sleeps, or works; what someone looks like; whether they have a partner or high-status job, and so on). Sometimes these judgments can remind you of a parent, family member, boss, childhood bully, or other judgmental figure from your life.

It evokes feelings of inadequacy. One way to spot a rule is by noticing what it evokes. Do you feel anxious, fearful, guilty, or ashamed? Do you feel suffocated, resentful, or frustrated? Even if a rule seems to be for your own good, the way it's presented tends to make you feel like you're failing.

It triggers a sense of urgency. Rules can land as threats, making you feel like you need to solve or fix things right away. Notice whether you feel inclined to engage in a "fixing" behavior in response, such as counting, tracking, planning, researching, or even just fixating on the situation at hand.

Note that a rule is harmful for its rigidity, delivery method, and attachment of "success" and "failure" to your worth. It's not about the subject matter. You can value health or fitness, for example, without buying into any rules about the "right" way to pursue health. You can value something without shaming yourself into achieving it.

We can't control what thoughts pop into our heads, but we can control how much significance we attach to them. What you water grows. The more emphasis you put on a punishing or judgmental thought, the more important it seems. The more you practice noticing harsh thoughts and intentionally shifting to more compassionate language, the easier it will become to notice when a thought is rooted in optimization rules, and therefore, not worth taking seriously.

According to ACT, one of the reasons humans suffer is that we become fused to our thoughts. We treat our most bothersome thoughts as super true and super important. When your inner critic feeds you an unhelpful thought like *I'm so lazy, I'll never amount to anything*, you might get upset because you take that thought as truth. In ACT, this is called *cognitive fusion*. Mental messages *seem* true, so they must *be* true. You can free yourself from this mental trap using a process called *cognitive defusion*, which involves detaching from your thoughts and realizing they are just random ideas. In fact, those ideas are just words, which are really just bits of noise in the mind.

Think about when you hear someone speaking a language you don't know. To you, it likely just sounds like noise. Even if they're saying something really awful, you probably don't feel any emotional reaction. The reason you get upset by words is because you learned to associate a particular meaning with those words. You can reverse engineer that association process and take power out of upsetting language by turning it back into a meaningless set of noises.

Practicing Cognitive Defusion

Think of words or phrases that have been used against you, either by bullies in your life or by your inner bully. Maybe you've been called sensitive, lazy, ugly, loud, dramatic, or stupid. Those words sting because of the meaning you've learned to attach to them. You've learned that those words *should* upset you.

At http://www.newharbinger.com/54063, you'll find an exercise designed to help you take power out of bothersome ideas, by reminding yourself that they are just random bits of noise. You'll identify a thought that bothers you and try these strategies to manipulate that thought:

- Introduce the thought with any of the following phrases: "My brain is telling me that…" "I'm having the thought that…" "The bully in my head keeps telling me…" followed by the thought. Reread it with the intro phrase and notice if it loses any power.

- Repeat the thought over and over until it sounds like babble. Start by saying it out loud twenty times in a row. If it's still bothersome after twenty repetitions, keep repeating until it loses power.

- Sing the thought to the tune of a song (try "Happy Birthday" or "Twinkle, Twinkle, Little Star").

- Write the thought backward (begin the sentence with the last word). Then, write it again but scramble all the letters and words around.

- Say the thought aloud several times in different silly voices.

After each strategy, you'll write about how it felt.

I used this activity to defuse from the thought *I'm so selfish*. For a long time, *selfish* was the worst thing I could be. I spent years trying to prove I was *not* selfish, compulsively denying my needs and agreeing to any request made of me. This didn't quiet the voice in my head that still told me I was selfish. Ironically, what made a difference wasn't convincing myself that I'm *not* selfish; it was realizing that "selfish" is just a word. It could hurt me only if I let it. If someone thought I was selfish, that was just their opinion, not the truth! Plus, so what if I *am* selfish? Why does that word get to have so much power over me, when I'm just an ordinary person trying to live my life? If you take the power out of words, then words don't hold power over you.

Even when you practice defusing from rules, pressures to optimize may still swirl around you. People in your life might continue glorifying discipline and productivity, and remnants of old rules may creep up. While you can't control whether these thoughts pop into your head, you can get better at recognizing them. Your thoughts aren't always a reflection of true, deep-down beliefs. If you're not sure whether a thought is harsh or compassionate, get curious. Ask yourself whether the message was framed as a command, or implied that you were good or bad. Sometimes, the message is well-intentioned but the voice is cruel. Try to rephrase the message to be more encouraging and compassionate.

If you're anything like my high-achieving clients, you may wonder why you should bother shifting to compassionate self-talk. Our culture emphasizes "no pain, no gain." You may believe that forcing yourself beyond your limits is the only way to improve. If you're kind to yourself, won't you just get complacent? While it may seem like the best way to get yourself to achieve is to ramp up the self-criticism, the opposite is actually true. The more you force yourself to bathe in shame and inadequacy, the stronger your desire becomes to *never* make another mistake. You might feel an urge to hide and fix, like you read about in chapter 2. Hiding and fixing might temporarily soothe you, but these strategies prevent you from taking risks or connecting with people because you worry that they might eventually see your vulnerabilities and flaws.

Self-compassion, not self-criticism, is the key to true growth. By showing yourself kindness even when you've screwed up, you can better understand emotions, learn from mistakes, and connect more deeply to yourself and other people. Buddhists believe that you have to care about yourself in order to fully care about others. In her groundbreaking book *Self-Compassion: The Proven Power of Being Kind to Yourself*, Dr. Kristin Neff (2015) blends Buddhist principles with concepts from Western psychology.

She explains, "If you are continually judging and criticizing yourself while trying to be kind to others, you are drawing artificial boundaries and distinctions that only lead to feelings of separation and isolation."

If you're constantly striving for perfection, you're situating yourself in a hierarchy where you must be better or worse than the people around you. How can you excel unless you're surpassing others? That's a recipe for insecurity, competitiveness, and disconnection. As we'll explore in the next chapter, our culture infuses wellness and hustle behaviors with morality, leading us to compare ourselves to one another and feel like we aren't measuring up. Yet your eating, fitness, and productivity do not make you any better or worse than anyone else—no matter what you were taught.

Being gentle toward yourself might feel strange or indulgent at first, but this attitude will support your ability to grow. Recognizing that you're *just a human*, and therefore flawed, can help you forgive yourself when you do end up doing something you regret. Rejecting optimization rules and embracing nuance will allow you to detach morality from your daily choices. You've been taught to hinge your self-worth on being optimal, but regardless of your achievement or output, you have inherent worth. No matter what those optimization rules try to tell you, there is no grading system for a life well lived.

CHAPTER 4

You're Not Special for Drinking Celery Juice

Every afternoon at 1:30 on the dot, I peed in a cup and tore open a foil packet containing an at-home ovulation testing strip. I'd set a timer for five minutes and then add a photo of the results to my fertility tracking app. When I saw a darkened test line, I sent a screenshot to my husband Jeremy, letting him know tonight we should "get busy." Forget about being in the mood; when the app said it was time to make a baby, we listened.

I'd been ambivalent about whether I wanted kids until just a few years prior. I spent my entire twenties terrified that if I missed a birth control pill, I'd instantly become pregnant. By my early thirties, I was still more of a "strong maybe" than a "hell yes." Still, I wanted it enough to try to make it happen, and with everyone around us popping out children left and right, we decided it was our time. Once I made the decision, it was like a switch flipped. I went from compulsively trying to avoid a pregnancy to compulsively trying to guarantee one. I thought about it nonstop. I read books, listened to podcasts, did manifestation exercises, diligently took prenatal vitamins, and figured out exactly which metrics to track. I wanted to optimize my mind and body for fertility. I'd do everything possible to have the healthiest and most successful pregnancy and childbirth. If I was going to do this, I was going to do it *right*.

Each month felt like I'd crammed nonstop to take an exam that I just kept failing. I racked my brain for where I'd gone wrong. Why had I been so singularly focused on building my career, wasting my most fertile years? Why hadn't I wanted this sooner? Aren't women supposed to just intuitively crave motherhood? Was I not energetically open enough to letting the universe grant me this gift? Was I tracking wrong? I must not be eating enough fish, kale, and walnuts. Maybe if I hadn't smoked so much weed or partied in my early twenties, I'd be more fertile now. Maybe if I'd done more yoga, gone to bed at more reasonable hours, and not been so set on defying traditional gender norms, I'd be pregnant by now. Even when part of me knew I was being irrational, another part of me believed my infertility was entirely my fault. I was just an overly indulgent, self-absorbed woman who thought I could have my cake and eat it too.

After fifteen months of this song and dance, Jeremy and I sat in straight-backed chairs facing our infertility specialist. I had procrastinated making the appointment, each month hopeful that *this* would be the month we finally nailed it. Eventually, I couldn't ignore the fissure forming in my fragile denial. This wasn't working. I needed a specialist to tell me what I was doing wrong so I could fix it. Several tests and procedures later, I was diagnosed with a diminished ovarian reserve. It turns out that no matter how meticulously we tracked, we had only ever had about a 3 percent chance of getting pregnant naturally. I was both devastated and momentarily relieved. Maybe it didn't matter what I'd done or not done. Maybe I wasn't making bad choices after all. Maybe this was something that had never been in my control in the first place.

That relief was quickly replaced by a new set of rules about how to be good or bad as a patient undergoing in vitro fertilization (IVF), which I learned was going to be my only real option for becoming pregnant. For as long as I could remember, I had absorbed infuriatingly contradictory information about what it meant to have a baby, and now that it wasn't happening the "right" way, I was surrounded by implications that I had done things wrong.

Undergoing IVF was like having a second full-time job—one that was exorbitantly expensive, time-consuming, and invasive, requiring both significant privilege and sacrifice. In order to be "good," I definitely couldn't complain about the needles, drugs, and procedures, the hormones and unpleasant side effects, or the crushing devastation when I did everything as instructed and it still didn't work. To be "good," I had to follow all of the rules and be vigilant, but also relax because stress is bad for fertility. I needed to be optimistic and keep my hopes up, but not too attached to a plan because it could take several cycles to get pregnant. Most of all, I was "good" if I stayed positive and chipper, and "bad" if I admitted I was deeply terrified I'd never meet my baby. People didn't want to handle my intensity; it was good to keep it under wraps.

My experience with infertility highlights the stark contrast between what we're told to do, how we're told to be, and what is actually possible. If you're good, you'll be rewarded and get what you want. If you're bad, you'll struggle and it will be your own fault. If things don't go your way, you must have done something wrong. We're given the message that there is *always* a right and wrong way to do things. Although reality doesn't necessarily reflect this, we continue to gravitate toward appraisals of our every move as good or bad, often to our own detriment.

The Good/Bad Trap

The human brain is pleased by categories. For most of our species' existence, it was vital to our survival to quickly parse out whether something (or someone) was good or bad, safe or unsafe. While it's useful to recognize whether an approaching beast is dangerous or harmless, or whether berries are safe to eat or poisonous, we get into hot water when we try to categorize *everything* according to this good/bad binary. When the messaging around us preys on this tendency to categorize, we end up framing every choice and characteristic as "good" or "bad." We begin to moralize ourselves, attaching judgments of good and bad to our habits, choices, thoughts, feelings—and our entire existence.

In the worlds of wellness and hustle, we constantly face opportunities to put ourselves into categories. Hustle culture teaches that it is "good" to spend one's time productively and "bad" to procrastinate or engage in activities that aren't goal directed. By these measures, you've been good if you've crossed off your entire to-do list for the day, and bad if you got distracted or lost motivation. You're supposed to ignore internal cues and ensure that everything you do is designed to generate wealth or optimize your health, fitness, and wellness. Spending time on things that serve no purpose besides being enjoyable is seen as self-indulgent, frivolous, a waste of time.

Every little decision can be categorized as good or bad, praiseworthy or guilt inducing, all the way down to what you eat for breakfast. When it comes to diet, we see this binary in how foods are labeled as good or bad, virtuous or sinful. Advertisements market calorie-dense foods as "indulgent." Products lower in sugar, fat, or carbs (depending on what's villainized at the time) are portrayed as "smart." Trader Joe's even brands their lower-calorie products with the label *Reduced Guilt*, implying that not only have the calories and fat content (and I'd add, the flavor and satisfaction) been reduced but also the *guilt* you'd be feeling if you committed the crime of eating a full-calorie bowl of macaroni and cheese. If you weren't aware that food has moral value before, you sure do now that you're buying something to reduce guilt!

Not only is there a "good" and "bad" way to eat, there are also constantly changing sets of recommendations about your overall health and wellness practices. One day it's good to dry brush and drink spirulina smoothies, the next day it's admirable to massage your face with a jade roller and drink celery juice. You have to avoid processed foods or plastic packaging (or both), depending on what's demonized that day. If you're doing the right things, you're showing the world your dedication to achieving well-being and happiness. You're responsible, inspiring, and somehow better than all the people who aren't doing these things.

A lot of binary thinking comes from the idea that what happens to you is the direct result of your effort. Diet culture preaches that you can control your body size and shape by controlling your food and physical activity. Wellness culture preaches that you can also control your health by controlling your food, physical activity, supplement intake, and participation in various wellness trends. Let's reiterate the truth: Even if everyone ate the exact same food and did the exact same physical activity, our bodies would still come in a wide variety of shapes and sizes (Matz and Frankel 2024), and would still have a wide variety of health outcomes. Even if everyone used the same productivity tools and strategies, we'd still each have different degrees of output.

The habits, behaviors, and images that are idealized as the morally correct way to be are also most accessible to people who already *have* a lot of those things. You need some degree of privilege to have the time and disposable income required to participate in most of these mandates. It's expensive to buy fresh, organic produce and stock up on the latest superfood (which, incidentally, is just a buzzword used to popularize a normal fruit, nut, or seed; items labeled as superfoods contain no nutritional properties that make them any different from other fruits, nuts, or seeds). It takes time—a luxury not afforded to many who work long hours, face long commutes, or don't have help with housework or childcare—to cook nutritious meals from scratch. Regular exercise takes time, physical ability, and a safe environment in which to be physically active, circumstances not everyone has.

Beauty standards promoted in Western culture are often centered around white, young, thin, cisgender, abled, and wealthy individuals. Body trends change with the decade, ensuring that if you achieve the ideal one day it will morph into something else the next. The skin-and-bones "heroin chic" aesthetic of the early 2000s gave way to the curvy, big booty ideal of the 2010s. Whatever is least attainable is held up as the goal. An obvious illustration of this is in a powerful industry targeting the one reality all human beings face: quite literally, the passage of time. The antiaging market was valued at $63 billion in 2022 and is projected to reach a value of more than $106 billion by 2030, according to a Vantage market research report (Hancock 2023).

Health, well-being, and standards of success are affected by far more than individual choices. Genetics, socioeconomic status, trauma and adverse childhood events, stress, experiences of stigma and discrimination, access to quality health care, mental health care, and preventative health care, exposure to environmental pollution, and numerous other factors contribute to whether someone achieves cultural standards of health or wealth (McGovern 2014). A large portion of health outcomes are determined by social factors, referred to as social determinants of health (SDoH). According to the World Health Organization, SDoH are the "conditions in which people are born, grow, live, work, and age…shaped by the distribution of money, power and resources at global, national and local levels." Nobody chooses the circumstances into which they are born, their biology or genetics, so the amount of influence someone has over their health is pretty minimal. In fact, individual behaviors make up only about 30 percent of what determines our health outcomes, and of that 30 percent, only about 10 percent is based on diet and exercise. The other 20 percent includes behaviors like alcohol consumption, substance use, tobacco, motor vehicle behavior, gun behavior, psychological coping behaviors, and sleep behavior (Hood et al. 2016).

Suffice it to say, you might be doing everything within your power to optimize and maximize your well-being, and still at best you'd only be influencing one-third of the factors involved. It's no wonder so many people feel like they're failing, when they've been instilled with the idea that they have more control over their outcomes than they actually do. Just as I believed I wasn't doing the right things to manifest a pregnancy, you might think that if you're not getting where you want to go, it's completely your fault. When you buy into the idea that you're in full control of your fate, you're being set up to attribute negative judgments to yourself when you fall short. Instead of recognizing mistakes, hardships, or unproductive days as natural human experiences, you learn to see them as signs that you're bad or morally inferior. You continue to seek answers from the very industries that taught you to feel bad about yourself in the first place.

Have you ever heard the diet-culture adage "You are what you eat"? The idea that your entire selfhood is dependent on your food choices says everything about our culture's association of self-control with moral goodness. The no-excuses mentality not only screams of privilege, it lacks nuance and disregards the variability of human experience, both from human to human and moment to moment. When you infuse morality into every little thing you do and call those things good or bad, that moral judgment can extend deeper into your overall self-perception. If it's good to go to bed early and bad to stay up late, then staying up late means you've done something bad. Beyond that, because you're doing something bad, your mind tells you that you *are* bad.

In cognitive behavioral theory, the tendency to think in good/bad binaries is often called all-or-nothing thinking (or black-and-white thinking). This type of thinking erases the complexity that comes with most situations, and contributes to a great deal of suffering for the thinker. When you're thinking logically, you likely know that a bedtime is morally neutral. Even if you don't really believe that your bedtime makes you superior or inferior to anyone else, your mind still tells you otherwise, making you feel like you've failed.

What Am I Moralizing?

You may have learned to attach morality to many of your habits and choices: how early you wake up, what you eat, how you spend your time and energy, or how much striving you're doing. Take a moment to consider your knee-jerk reactions to the following behaviors. Does your brain tell you they're good, bad, or neutral? Be honest; remember this is only to help you recognize the false morality you've been instilled with.

- Staying up until two a.m. playing video games
- Going to the gym after work each day
- Answering work emails as soon as they hit your inbox
- Ordering takeout five times in one week
- Waking up at six a.m. to read nonfiction before work
- Letting dishes pile up in the sink for a few days before washing them
- Making your own nut butters and jams from scratch
- Doing a ten-step skincare routine each evening

It's understandable to have an automatic judgment of these behaviors even if logically you don't think any are inherently good or bad. It may help to remind yourself that there is no universal authority on what makes a bedtime, or any other habit, good or bad. Get curious about whether it's helpful to categorize your behavior in such a binary way. Perhaps underneath the judgment you can learn something about yourself. Do you face an unwanted consequence when you go to bed at two in the morning? If you think you would benefit from making a change to your bedtime (or any other habit), perhaps you can offer yourself encouragement about changing that behavior without attaching it to a moral category. Instead of telling yourself that one habit is good and the other bad, you can simply observe that one habit is more helpful to you in a given circumstance.

When you feel negative toward yourself, you might draw negative conclusions about yourself based on that feeling. Called emotional reasoning, this is another way your mind can contribute to suffering, where what you're feeling seems true even when logically you know it isn't. Every month I had a negative pregnancy test, I felt like a failure. Through emotional reasoning, I believed that feeling like a failure meant I *was* a failure. As I often remind clients (and myself), feelings aren't facts, and thoughts aren't truth with a capital T. Yet when thoughts and feelings seem true, they can be really hard to recognize as just thoughts and feelings, temporary and transient inner experiences that may or may not reflect anything useful about ourselves or the world. This is when it can be helpful to use those cognitive defusion practices from chapter 3 to distance yourself from the thought and evaluate it as just a random group of words passing through your mind, not necessarily worth taking seriously. The same goes with feelings. You can feel a temporary set of sensations without it meaning that those sensations define you.

Taking a curious, nonjudgmental attitude toward your habits and decisions can help you meet yourself with greater clarity, so that you can actually grow. It's not usually helpful to beat yourself up for something that has already happened, since you can't change the past. If you can get curious about the outcome of a past decision, you can discover whether you want to repeat that behavior or whether it would be more valuable to choose something different. Self-compassion doesn't make you self-indulgent. I've never seen someone effectively shame themself into growth, but I have seen a lot of people grow through kindly encouraging themselves.

When you judge yourself as bad for something, whether big or small, pause and think critically about that judgment. Do you truly believe that you're a bad person, or is it more accurate to say that you feel guilt or remorse over whatever you just said or did? Is your guilt a reflection of the fact that you did something that conflicted with your values and went against the type of person you want to be? For example, did you snap at your partner, and now you feel guilty because you value kindness, and that wasn't so kind? Or is your guilt a conditioned response to what society taught you to care about, but deep down you know it doesn't really matter? For example, maybe you had a friend visiting and you chose to skip your morning workout to have breakfast with them. Is your guilt truly an indication that you did something morally reprehensible, or is it a response to being taught you're supposed to exercise every day?

If you can develop a more neutral self-perception and see yourself as just human, not good or bad, you can treat each moment as a new moment in which to decide how to behave. In any given moment you have infinite options for where to put your focus and resources. If you can stop fixating on which choice is right and which is wrong, and stop attaching good and bad judgments to yourself in the process, you have flexibility to do whatever is authentic to you in that particular moment, knowing it can change across time and circumstances. The best you can do is consider how you wish to behave in the current situation, and attempt to behave that way, knowing sometimes you'll stray or be unable to follow through despite good intentions.

Nobody deserves to be defined by how they feel in a given moment, how much they produce, or what accolades they achieve. Your health and wellness practices don't make you better or worse than anyone, nor do your behaviors around work and productivity. You aren't what you eat. You aren't your bedtime, bank account, or job title. You aren't even your personality traits, which can intensify or diminish based on mood, energy, and circumstances. We're living organisms, not machines. I have never actually valued someone more because they ordered a kale salad or worked eighty hours in a week. Most of us value our loved ones simply for being themselves, not for what they produce or achieve. True well-being doesn't come from how well a person is "optimizing" according to arbitrary, narrow, and elitist standards. True well-being is subjective and context dependent. What adds meaning to your life might be different from what adds meaning to mine, and might change over time. Regardless, your worth as a living being does not increase or decrease for any reason.

At our core, all humans want to matter. Mattering is "an ideal state of affairs consisting of two complementary psychological experiences: feeling valued and adding value" (Prilleltensky 2019). You can feel valued by your own self, by others, and by your community. You can also add value to your own self, others, or your community. These are important elements of feeling fulfilled and whole. When you receive the message, intended or not, that you matter only if you fulfill some set of metrics, you begin chasing things that don't mean anything significant to you or to the people around you. You come up feeling empty and disconnected from both yourself and the important people in your life. On the other hand, if you surround yourself with people who don't emphasize empty metrics and value you for the same things you value in yourself, you can fulfill this need for mattering.

Having a clear sense of your values, or the qualities and characteristics you wish to embody in your daily life, will help you fulfill your need for mattering. When you fulfill your need to matter, you build a strong and stable self-worth. That means your self-worth won't depend on your mood and won't get shattered if you make a mistake or experience a setback. Understanding what matters to you at a deeper level will help you make choices that aren't based on external measures or desire for approval. Interestingly, when you live according to your values, you also find yourself connecting more deeply with people who share and appreciate those values. Chapter 5 will focus on the process of figuring out your personal values, so you can reorient yourself toward them as you continue to move through life. Your values will guide you not with moral judgment or labels of "good" and "bad," but with clarity and compassion.

Taking Back the Steering Wheel

PART 2

CHAPTER 5

Redefining Your Values

Wellness and hustle cultures promote extrinsic motivation, which involves doing things to satisfy an external force or obtain external reward (like praise, a good grade, or a paycheck). Extrinsic motivation is woven into the fabric of our culture, from the classroom to the boardroom. It starts from a young age. Children are rewarded with a weekly allowance in exchange for household tasks. They earn an A-plus in the classroom and stickers on a behavior chart. At first, it's exciting for a six-year-old to see stickers filling their chart. Eventually, it's not so special. Plus, they learn that the reason to act a certain way is to get a reward. Although extrinsic motivation may work in the short run, its effects wear off over time.

On the other hand, when someone is intrinsically motivated, they pursue the inner satisfaction of successfully completing a project, mastering a skill, or knowing they added value to their family or community. The child clears the dinner table not to earn a gold star, but to get the internal reward of feeling like a helpful and important member of the family. This is a path toward mattering, that sense of belongingness that is so important for building self-worth. Feeling valued both by oneself and others helps a child build resilience in the face of wellness and hustle messaging.

Many of us are afraid that without extrinsic motivation keeping us accountable we'll never accomplish anything. However, the research paints a different picture. Research on employee motivation indicates that when people are intrinsically motivated, they are more engaged in their work and more willing to take on responsibilities (Edirisooriya 2014; Cho and Perry 2012; Grant 2008). Having a strong sense of intrinsic motivation is associated with greater job satisfaction, more persistence, and lower likelihood of quitting (Cho and Perry 2012). In the classroom, using external motivators to get kids to complete tasks may even backfire. Research has shown that grades and rewards can hinder the learning process (Baranek 1996).

Meanwhile, when a student is intrinsically motivated, they learn faster and actually want to learn because they enjoy the experience of growing and advancing.

On the reality television show *Survivor*, participants compete in challenges to win rewards like food, tools to improve camp life, or immunity from being voted out of the game. During a particularly grueling physical challenge, one competitor, a self-proclaimed couch potato with little athletic prowess, struggled on the obstacle course while her competitors nimbly ran, climbed, and swam their way through. Her performance was the clear reason her tribe lost the challenge that day. Yet afterward, rather than slink away in shame, she continued running the course, although the prize was already claimed. When she finally got to the end, the emotion on her face was undeniable. It was clear that for her, finishing the challenge was not about external reward or the external validation of her teammates; it was about proving something to herself. This is the power of intrinsic motivation; it allows us to prove ourselves far more capable than we could ever imagine.

Like most things in life, motivation isn't all-or-nothing. No matter how internally driven you are, you probably still need a paycheck in exchange for your work. No matter how satisfied you feel by a job well done, you still need others to acknowledge your contributions sometimes. However, when extrinsic rewards are overemphasized, we end up pursuing things that may not be personally meaningful. When you pursue goals that you find genuinely fulfilling, not just ones you think you *should* pursue, you tend to stick with them even when they're hard. The key is figuring out what's important enough that you'll still care about it even with no trophy at the end. You can do this by exploring which of your choices are intrinsically driven.

Imagine you have two friends, Graciela and Liz, who both wake up at the crack of dawn to go running. Graciela took up running in college and enjoys the consistency it provides to her weekly routines. She has since run two marathons and is amazed by her body's ability to build endurance for long distances. Running makes her feel strong and powerful. Although she isn't always in the mood to run, Graciela still pushes herself because she likes how she feels afterward. Running gives her an energy boost that she carries with her throughout the rest of her day. She isn't rigid about it; on mornings when she could use more rest, she skips her run. For Graciela, running enhances her quality of life.

Liz, on the other hand, dreads her morning runs. Liz took up running to try to lose weight after having her second child. Now, her husband gets the kids ready for school each morning while she clips on a fitness tracker and pushes herself along, silently calculating how many calories she needs to burn to compensate for the chicken nuggets she ate off her toddler's plate the night before. Liz hates running, and hates that to fit it into her day she has to miss quality time with her family. She wishes she could eat breakfast with her kids; she can picture her daughter giggling at her husband's silly dance while he flips pancakes, and feels a pang of sadness for missing these precious moments. Still, Liz believes that running is the better choice, and the price she must pay for her postpartum body.

Although Graciela and Liz run the same distances with the same frequency, their relationships with running could not be more different. Graciela's relationship with running is mostly positive, as she is motivated by her values. Liz runs as an attempt to control her body size. She is motivated not by her own values, but by externally imposed ones. In fact, one of the reasons Liz resents her morning run is that it takes her away from something that she *does* value—the chance to spend quality time with her loved ones.

From the outside, nobody can tell whether you're running (or doing anything else) because of intrinsic motivation or because of external pressures and expectations. Only you can know the truth, and the truth lies in your values. Values are the qualities that you deem as most important to you. These are the characteristics you strive to embody in everyday life. One way to uncover your values is to think about how you'd want people to describe you at your funeral—caring, adventurous, thoughtful, trustworthy, and so forth. Some of the words that come to mind for how I hope people will remember me are "warm," "authentic," and "supportive." What comes to mind for you is yours alone—no right or wrong.

Another way to clarify values is to consider experiences that bring you a sense of purpose or fulfillment, such as love, learning, friendship, nature, or spiritual growth. You can uncover your values by paying attention to what lights you up. The things that excite you aren't random; they reflect your unique passions. A deep desire to travel and try new things could stem from valuing variety, adventure, or curiosity. Similarly, the things that rile you might upset you because they conflict with your values. Anger when learning of war or upheaval could point to values of peace, harmony, or cooperation.

A value is a direction, not a destination. If you value kindness, you don't just behave kindly once and you're done. Kindness is the path you're seeking to follow every day. If you accidentally say or do something unkind, you realize that you strayed off the path and recommit. Valuing kindness doesn't mean you do it perfectly; it means committing to being kind over and over again. Each new moment presents you with a new opportunity to behave kindly.

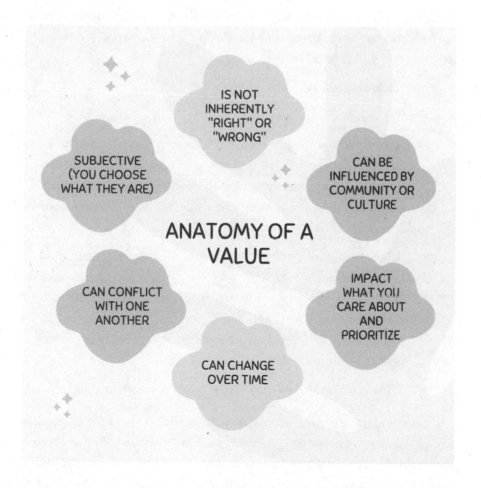

ANATOMY OF A VALUE

IS NOT INHERENTLY "RIGHT" OR "WRONG"

CAN BE INFLUENCED BY COMMUNITY OR CULTURE

SUBJECTIVE (YOU CHOOSE WHAT THEY ARE)

CAN CONFLICT WITH ONE ANOTHER

IMPACT WHAT YOU CARE ABOUT AND PRIORITIZE

CAN CHANGE OVER TIME

When you're behaving in alignment with your values, you tend to feel more satisfied with your behavior than when you're acting in ways that go against your values. The tricky part for those of us stuck in toxic striving is that we focus so much on living in accordance with whatever we hope will get us approval or acceptance from others that we don't always know what feels personally meaningful. A key aspect of what makes something a value is that it is subjective, meaning there are no values that are universally correct or incorrect. Nobody else gets to tell you what you value or how much something matters to you.

What Do You Stand For?

This exercise is designed to help you clarify which values you most want to embody and represent. Using your journal, write about a time you behaved in a way that you're proud of.

- What did you say or do?

- Was it difficult for you to act that way? Why or why not?

- How would you describe your behavior in that scenario? (For example, did you behave in a way that was courageous, generous, authentic, assertive, friendly, patient, loyal, intelligent, mature? You can use more than one word to describe your behavior).

- What is something you find rewarding, or something you would be upset about if you were told you could never do it? (For example, traveling, spending time in nature, spending time with particular friends or loved ones, painting, listening to music, participating in a religious or spiritual event, being a parent, hosting a celebration)

- What is it that makes those experiences rewarding to you?

Now read the following list of values. Circle five or six of the words that resonate with you as personally meaningful. They may be words that capture the significance of the experiences you described above. If you find it meaningful to spend time with your partner, perhaps you value family, connection, or love. If you find it meaningful to draw or paint, perhaps you value creativity, self-expression, beauty, or art. If you identify with any values that aren't on this list, write them in the spaces at the end.

Adventure	Fitness	Organization
Achievement	Freedom	Patience
Acceptance	Friendship	Peace
Assertiveness	Fun	Perseverance
Authenticity	Generosity	Presence
Autonomy	Gratitude	Reliability
Beauty	Health	Resilience
Boldness	Honesty	Respect
Charisma	Hope	Responsibility
Community	Humor	Self-awareness
Compassion	Inclusivity	Self-development
Connection	Integrity	Spirituality
Cooperation	Intentionality	Stability
Courage	Intimacy	Strength
Creativity	Justice	Supportiveness
Critical thinking	Kindness	Tolerance
Curiosity	Leadership	Trustworthiness
Dedication	Learning	Warmth
Discipline	Logic	Variety
Emotional maturity	Love	Other:
Fairness	Loyalty	Other:
Faith	Nature	Other:
Family	Open-mindedness	Other:
Flexibility	Optimism	

Now, list all five or six of the values you identified, big and bold, all in one place.

What If You Value Health or Hustle?

Maybe your tendency for striving is not just the result of your condition-ing. You may reflect and discover that yes, you *do* value achievement. The same can be true for health or fitness. Yet even if you find that deep down, you value some of the same things that the culture at large pro-motes, you may not value them in the same *ways*. Consider not only what you value, but how you define those values.

For example, wellness and diet culture define "health" in a specific way: eating exclusively nutrient-dense foods, getting physical activity, and maintaining a body free of disease and signs of aging. While nutri-ents and physical activity can absolutely enhance someone's life, that doesn't mean that anyone is obligated to define health in these terms— or even to value health at all! Maybe you subscribe to a definition of health that includes mental health, healthy relationships, or financial or spiritual health. Maybe a healthy life for you involves safe sex, wearing a seatbelt, and managing stress. Just because wellness culture twists health to be only about a specific set of metrics (including many factors not in our control), that doesn't mean these are the *only* ways to honor health.

Similarly, if you genuinely value productivity, discipline, or achieve-ment, how do you define these concepts? Hustle culture defines them as waking up early, jam-packing your schedule, and working long hours. Maybe for you, productivity means regularly creating things that con-tribute to a larger purpose. Maybe you value discipline, but not in the form of denying yourself pleasure. Perhaps for you, achievement involves tapping into that adaptive form of perfectionism we explored in chapter 2. Many people value learning and self-development. Hustle culture dis-torts these into harsh mandates, but they do not have to be this way.

The bottom line is that only *you* get to decide what you value, and how you choose to honor your values each day.

Now that you're aware of what matters to you, it may feel like self-betrayal to continue pursuing externally imposed values over your own. However, prioritizing your values is not always easy. Rejecting societal stan-dards can make you more vulnerable to stigma or judgment. There isn't a pain-free choice. It's up to you to decide which pain is most worth tolerating—the pain of rejection by some people (in exchange for the meaningfulness of acting authentically), or the pain of forcing yourself to comply with outside standards (in exchange for the comfort and safety of fitting in). Remember that you're not the problem. Broken systems, unhelpful conditioning, and a harsh inner critic are the real problems, as they keep you chasing moving targets at the expense of your well-being.

There is hope; systems can change, but usually not overnight. Throughout history, our species has demonstrated the ability to progress beyond an existing set of ideals. The more each of us becomes aware of unrealistic standards, the more we can actively reject them. We can stop trying to turn ourselves into a bunch of smooth, glowy, firm-bodied productivity robots. We can stop glorifying discipline and normalizing burnout. Starting with our own small worlds, we can change what is held up as ideal. By surrounding ourselves with others who are also committed to rejecting harmful ideals, and sharing openly about what we truly care about, we can appreciate one another's differences. Over time, we can create a world that accepts and even celebrates the diversity of brains, bodies, and personalities that naturally exists across our species.

Yet even as we shift culturally, it would be unrealistic to expect a world where nobody struggles. Intrusive and automatic thoughts, stressors, hassles, and discomfort are simply realities of being alive. Even the most privileged among us will eventually experience hardship, if only through the passing of time. Brains will lose sharpness, bodies will lose function, and loved ones will pass away. This isn't news to most of us, but we still have a hard time accepting it. Instead, we lose ourselves in striving for control, subconsciously believing that if we try hard enough, we can achieve a comfortable, pain-free life.

While there's no secret formula for a happy, easy life, things aren't completely hopeless. Once you recognize that you can't control whether you experience hardship or pain, nor can you control what you feel inside, you can practice accepting what you cannot control. Accepting doesn't mean you like it or want it (who *wants* life to be hard?) but it means you're going to stop struggling against it since that struggle is just a waste of energy. The more you free up the energy you were using to try to control things you couldn't control, you can direct that energy toward what you *can* control: your behavior. This is where having a clear sense of your values comes into play.

If all you can control is your behavior, you probably want to be intentional about that behavior. Don't underestimate how much your behavior impacts not only your own quality of life but also the lives of the people around you. While you can't control whether something causes you to feel frustrated, you can control how you behave in response to that event and the feeling of frustration that was evoked. You choose whether you respond by sulking, lashing out, storming out of the room, or taking a few deep breaths and reflecting on the situation. While you can't choose how another person treats you, you can choose how you treat them. If someone is disrespectful toward you, it's up to you whether you get passive-aggressive, insult them, say nothing, assert a boundary, or walk away. You can't control the messed-up parts of society, but you can control how you engage with society. If you hold a value that differs from what society promotes (for instance, valuing authenticity in a world that rewards conformity), you can still make an impact on your own social circle and community by staying true to your personal values. This might even give others permission to do the same, having a ripple effect over time. In any situation, consider your options and choose the action that is most likely to make you proud of yourself afterward. Usually, your values will clue you in.

Your values serve as a sort of road map, guiding you toward the type of person you wish to be and the type of life you wish to lead. You can use them to set short-term and long-term goals for yourself. If you value family, perhaps a values-aligned goal would be to connect with a loved one once per week. When you consider how to behave in a given situation, you can turn to your values for the answer. What will make you proud of yourself looking back on this situation? What might you regret? Remember, it's not about acting perfectly; it's about making an effort to be the type of person you want to be. Take a moment to think about something you've already done this week that aligned with your values. It can be simple, like giving up your seat for another passenger on the bus. Then, consider how you can commit to more actions this week that align with your values. You can even create a ritual, each evening taking a moment to consider one thing you did

What Can You Control?

Things you CAN'T control

✖ Which thoughts come into your mind

✖ Which feelings arise

✖ What happens to you

✖ Other people (what they say, feel, think, or do)

Things you CAN control

✔ How much attention or importance you give your thoughts

✔ How you cope with feelings

✔ How you respond to what happens to you

✔ Your own behavior

that day (or one thing you wish to do tomorrow) that aligns with your values.

Doing the values-aligned thing is not always pleasant or enjoyable. Graciela mostly enjoys running, but that doesn't mean she enjoys every single second of it. She commits to it because she values the benefits it adds to her life. You may value patience, but that doesn't mean it will be easy to close your eyes and take a deep breath instead of snapping when your coworker asks, for the twentieth time, when you're going to have the report ready. When you look back on each day through the lens of "Was I living out my values today?" you'll start to practice validating yourself. In other words, you'll recognize when you're acting with purpose and give yourself credit where credit is due. You value authenticity and you were open with your friend about something she said that hurt your feelings? Give yourself a mental pat on the back! You value kindness and you rushed to open the door for someone who had their hands full? Time to pop that imaginary champagne!

Sure, we all still need external validation sometimes. The need to be seen, recognized, and valued by others is an important one. However, it is only half the equation, and the other half comes from within. When you develop a habit of internally validating, you become less dependent on the approval of others. Even if nobody else notices or praises you for it, *you* can still feel proud of yourself.

Acting in alignment with your values can make you vulnerable, especially in situations where other people don't share those values. Not everyone in your life will agree with your choices. You'll get pushback from people who are used to you doing what they want you to do. You'll also encounter that inner critic in your own mind, telling you that you're selfish, lazy, or letting yourself go for doing anything that isn't disciplined or productive. Yet while some will judge you for your values, others will appreciate you for them.

Most importantly, *you* will appreciate yourself more. Instead of asking *What would so-and-so want me to do here?*, you can practice asking *What would my values tell me to do here?* At the end of the day, you're on this planet to live, and that means living a full, rich, satisfying life—not just placating everyone around you while secretly feeling empty and exhausted. You're allowed to experience the full spectrum of feelings, thoughts, needs, cravings, and desires that arise within you.

In fact, when you truly believe this, you can even learn from those internal experiences. Maybe your cravings or instincts are telling you what you need, or pointing to an area where you've been feeling deprived. When you give yourself unconditional permission to exist as a messy human being and not a machine to optimize or control, your body and mind can work together in greater harmony. If what you resist persists, then when you stop resisting, those bothersome thoughts, feelings, and desires can simply run their course instead of plaguing you. In the next chapter, you'll explore the role of deprivation in your life, and learn to heal through unconditional permission to honor your physical, emotional, and spiritual needs with compassion.

CHAPTER 6

Unconditional Permission to Be Human

In high school, Allie was one of the only kids in class who actually studied during study hall. While her classmates passed notes, gossiped, or decorated their notebook covers, Allie sat up front and dutifully spent the hour puzzling over math homework or reading the assigned text for English lit. Allie regularly earned high grades, but she was sure that if she didn't force herself to study so hard, she'd fall behind. Each evening as she finished her homework, Allie watched her mom come home and pop in an aerobics tape. She would tell Allie, "If I don't exercise right when I get home, I'll never find the willpower to do it!" As an adult, Allie took a similar approach to exercise. She signed up for spin class the night before, entering a credit card to reserve her spot so she wouldn't be tempted to bail.

Willpower always seemed fleeting. She'd muster just enough to stick with a habit for a short while, and then it would vanish. On Sundays, she'd make five identical lunches for the week ahead, until one weekend she just *couldn't*. Then she'd berate herself for ordering takeout, and vow to get back into her meal prep routine the next weekend. The Herculean effort she put into maintaining a healthy and productive routine felt essential to her success. Everywhere she went, she was reminded that without willpower, she'd never accomplish what she needed to do each day. Willpower seemed like a magical resource that was quickly depleted; when the willpower burned out, so did she.

As a culture, we've come to glorify denial of our basic needs as "discipline" or "willpower." While the concept of deprivation has been glorified in many cultures throughout history, it has taken on new life in recent centuries. Particularly, in Western countries founded on puritanical, white supremacist beliefs, the idea that depriving oneself somehow made one superior was woven into the fabric of society. That mindset has trickled down over generations to color what we extol as virtuous behavior, and what is seen as lazy or gluttonous. Combine this with the Western-glorified idea that anyone can pull themselves up by the bootstraps and it's no surprise that when something is hard to sustain, we blame ourselves. If you're not able to *just do it*, the problem must be a personal deficiency. Even as the standards we strive for shift across decades and centuries, the glorification of "hustling" remains a constant throughline (Petersen 2020; Harrison 2019; Ravenelle 2019).

Historian Natalia Mehlman Petrzela (2022) describes how harnessing willpower for healthy habits has become a shared priority across groups—liberal or conservative, religious or agnostic—that disagree on most other matters. She writes, "Across the political and cultural spectrum, Americans have come to rare agreement that claiming agency over one's well-being, body and mind, is crucial to a life well lived." When someone has achieved success in the eyes of society, they may acknowledge opportunities or privileges that helped them reach these heights. However, they almost always will also credit their sheer will. They will mention sacrifice, discipline, how they worked hard and didn't make excuses.

Living from a "no excuses" mentality means operating in extremes. When you're on your game, you feel superhuman. When you inevitably crash, you can't figure out where you went wrong. After all, you were sticking with those habits, for days or even weeks on end! So why did you get off track, and how can you ensure it never happens again? Clinging harder to routines or searching for more effective productivity tools can seem like the solutions, but in reality, no living organism can sustain nonstop productivity. We all crash and burn eventually.

In *Can't Even: How Millennials Became the Burnout Generation*, journalist Anne Helen Petersen (2020) describes burnout as "the flattening of life into one never-ending to-do list, and the feeling that you've optimized yourself into a work robot that happens to have bodily functions, which you do your very best to ignore." The swing from *totally crushing it* to *catatonic on the couch* can feel dramatic, as if your machinery suddenly short-circuited. People often think the antidote to crashing is to just optimize harder, so they double down on their wellness or hustle routines. Until ultimately, the pendulum swings back in the other direction, and they hit burnout once again. This tendency reminds me of a common disordered eating pattern called the *restrict-binge cycle*.

I know it well because I've lived it. For years, I believed I had a night-time snacking problem. Really, it was a binge-eating problem. Most days, I ate a breakfast of an egg-white omelet and whole-wheat toast. Lunch was a salad with protein. I snacked on almonds and apples. Dinner was usually some form of protein, vegetables, and brown rice. I didn't consider myself a dieter; I just tried to eat healthy. People often praised my habits and asked me for recipes and advice.

What they didn't know was that every night, an hour or two after my healthy dinner, I would ravage my cabinets in search of dessert. I didn't let myself buy anything that wasn't healthified, so dessert was usually some messy concoction of monk fruit–sweetened "ice cream" topped with almond butter, dark chocolate, or if I was really in a pinch, crushed protein bars. Then I'd want savory, spreading cream cheese on crackers until I'd eaten the whole box. Then I'd go back to another sweet concoction, eating until I was in pain and vowing that tomorrow I'd have more self-control. I did this on repeat for nearly a decade. Daytime: egg whites, salads, almonds, tofu. Nighttime: fiend for sugar and salt until I was sick. I believed I couldn't be trusted with the foods I craved, like potato chips or brownies. After all, look how I behaved with low-sugar ice cream!

I was sure my problem was one of willpower. But despite popular belief, the real reason that most people can't stick to a restrictive way of eating for long has nothing to do with how badly they want it. It's simply biology. Bodies are wired to get their needs met and maintain homeostasis; when your body gets off balance, it seeks to return to balance. It sends hunger signals when it needs fuel, and fullness signals when it's gotten enough. When its core temperature gets too low, it makes you shiver, sending signals that make you want to put on a sweater. When your bladder gets too full, your body signals an urgency to pee. When we don't respond to those signals, the body resorts to more drastic measures. When chronically sleep deprived, you eventually crash hard. When chronically deprived of food, you eventually binge hard.

There's a reason most people don't binge on carrots or chicken breast. When a body is deprived, it thinks there's a famine. It doesn't know *why* you're eating too little—it just knows you're not eating enough. Your body tries to remedy the deficit by driving you toward foods that will break down into energy as quickly as possible—foods high in sugar or carbohydrates. Maybe you get that chance to compensate when you find yourself in a situation where more forbidden food is around, like a restaurant or vacation. Other times, you reach a breaking point and buy or order those off-limits foods. Then you feel guilty for caving, and tighten the reins to make up for it. And so, the restrict-binge cycle repeats itself.

Humans are, in some ways, sophisticated animals. We don't just have instincts; we also have emotions, thoughts, and memories. We develop complex associations between events and experiences in ways that other animals don't. While your dog may be content eating the same meal on repeat for its entire life, you probably won't be. Humans experience cravings and desires. Some are based on physical needs, like craving fresh fruits or vegetables when you haven't had any for a while, and some are emotional, like desiring a warm slice of your mom's homemade pie during the holidays. It's not always enough to fuel ourselves—we also need to feel psychologically satisfied by what we've eaten. In this regard, your body senses deprivation both when you're not eating enough food, and when you're not eating enough variety of food.

When we aren't satisfied, we often have cravings that are psychological and emotional in nature, rather than purely biological. You may technically be eating enough food, and you may eat whatever foods you want, so you're not deprived of calories or variety, but you could still feel a sense of psychological deprivation if you're placing shame on yourself around eating. For instance, maybe you scoop yourself a bowl of premium ice cream, but while eating it, you say things to yourself like *I shouldn't have this* or *I can only have one bowl*. That guilt prevents you from reaching satisfaction, so psychologically, it registers as if you didn't eat it at all. You still come away feeling deprived, but confused. It feels like you can never get enough, even if you're physically full. This is often where people falsely diagnose themselves with food addiction, when what's really happening is that they are psychologically deprived.

Just as limiting foods leads to out-of-control eating, restricting emotions can have a similar effect. The more you resist the expression or acknowledgment of a particular emotion, the more out-of-control and intense that emotion becomes. Early in my career, I worked in a chemical dependency treatment center for men recovering from opioid addiction. Much of what my clients and I focused on was learning how to move through tough emotions without using impulsive or self-destructive behaviors. One afternoon, I sat in my weekly therapy session with Tom, a sixty-year-old man who was newly sober. He had just been dumped by his long-term girlfriend, but he insisted it was no big deal. He was fine. I said gently, "You know, it's okay if you're not fine; heartbreak kind of sucks." Suddenly, he began crying; big sobs shook his entire body. The tears surprised us both. As this stoic man wept, he kept repeating, "It hurts *so* bad... it hurts *so* bad."

Opioids are such powerful painkillers that they can numb even the slightest discomfort. When you're used to replacing any pain with a constant drip of pleasure, difficult emotions aren't just difficult; they're pure torture. Sure enough, at that first ping of sadness, Tom felt a craving rush back in. He was certain that if he weren't in the safety of our treatment program he'd be relapsing that night. To Tom's credit, he stuck it out. With practice, supportive pharmacotherapy, and lifestyle changes, he learned how to tolerate unpleasant emotions and regulate himself without using drugs. Yet every time he felt something painful, his first reaction was a desire to numb.

In *Wherever You Go, There You Are*, Jon Kabat-Zinn (2005) explains that "you can't stop the waves, but you can learn to surf." You can't prevent the challenging moments, but you can learn to move through them without getting swept away. You're being knocked around by the current when you're on that pendulum of restrict, binge, restrict again only to binge again. You're also getting knocked around when you swing from bottling emotions to getting overwhelmed, back to trying to bottle up even harder, only to eventually explode. At the whims of the current, you're trapped in a cycle of fear, overcontrol, and burnout. There is an antidote to these extremes; there exists a surfboard you can climb upon that carries you over the waves of human experience. It might seem counterintuitive at first, but stick with me here: you learn to ride the waves by giving yourself what the authors of *Intuitive Eating* call unconditional permission (Tribole and Resch 2020).

With food, unconditional permission means allowing yourself to eat without limits, until your body begins to feel less frantic. That means allowing yourself not just to eat whatever appeals to you, but to have as much of those foods as your body desires, as frequently as your body desires. Your body eventually begins to trust that it will get what it's seeking, and that food won't be taken away again. The forbidden fruit is always the sweetest. As soon as you put limitations on something, it becomes all-consuming. When you remove limitations, it becomes ordinary. If you can eat french fries, pizza, or ice cream anytime you want, those foods soon lose their luster. It's the scarcity mindset that makes something irresistible. Moving from scarcity to abundance allows you to feel safe and calm.

The same process can apply to emotions. When you stop trying to *not* feel an unwanted emotion, that emotion may still be unpleasant, but it eventually becomes less scary. By exposing yourself to that emotion without trying to get rid of it, you learn how to experience it fully and then watch it fade away or morph into the next emotion. Don't get me wrong; it can feel downright terrifying to stop fighting for control. I can't tell you how many times I've seen people of all different ages and backgrounds doing everything in their power to *not* cry. People fear that if they let themselves cry, they will never stop. Or, if they let themselves cry they won't be able to tolerate the flood of emotions that surfaces. Fighting the release only makes it that much more unbearable. In reality, any emotion predictably peaks and then subsides. It's only when we mess with it by fueling it with unhelpful thoughts or engaging in control efforts that an emotion tortures us indefinitely.

Harvard neuroscientist Jill Bolte Taylor (2008) formulated the ninety-second rule. When you have a reaction to something in your environment (for example, a flash of anger when someone cuts you off in traffic), the chemical process that happens in your body lasts a total of ninety seconds. If the emotion continues after that, it's likely that the response is being restimulated by your thoughts or continued exposure to the stimulus that triggered it. If you can simply watch the process happen, and allow it to run from start to finish without prolonging it through efforts to make it go away, you might actually notice the intensity subside after less than two minutes. Sure, you may then have a similar feeling shortly after, but then *that* emotional response will run its course if you don't interfere. Like anything we try to avoid or control, the stimulus loses its power once it's given unconditional permission to be there.

Habituation: The First Bite Is the Most Delicious

It can be downright terrifying to give yourself unconditional permission to eat, rest, feel feelings, or allow any natural experiences you've previously tried to overcontrol. There is often a fear that once you start allowing yourself to eat potato chips anytime you want, you'll be unable to stop. You'll eat them on repeat 24/7 for the rest of time. While this might happen at first, it eventually goes away, thanks to a behavioral principle called habituation.

Habituation is what happens when the more frequently you're presented with a stimulus, the less intense your response becomes. With food, enjoyment is tied to novelty. The first bite is the newest and most delicious. Food lights up pleasure centers in the brain at first, but over time that response will diminish. Each bite is less exciting than the last. Think about how that first lick of an ice cream cone is the most enjoyable. With each subsequent lick, you get used to it and the reward value diminishes.

The intensity of your response to a food can also be tied to rules or beliefs you have about that food. Research shows that people rate food as more pleasurable and have a harder time stopping when full if they have been dieting, or deprived of that food (Epstein et al. 2003; Cameron et al. 2014; Hagan and Moss 1997). If a food is laced with rules, guilt, judgment, or scarcity, it never loses its allure, even if you keep eating and eating it. When you're approaching food from a place of psychological (or physical) deprivation, you're chronically unsatisfied. That's why people who try to eliminate or limit certain foods often feel addicted to those foods. Once someone has been given consistent unconditional permission to eat, they'll eat something if they're hungry or it appeals to them, and leave it if it doesn't.

Consider other examples of habituation you may be familiar with beyond food. The first time you kiss a new romantic partner, you might feel intensely over-the-moon happy. Ten years into a relationship, when you kiss that same partner, it might be nice, but it won't have the same level of pleasure and intensity that it did early in the relationship. After that honeymoon phase wears off, we habituate to the stimulus of our partner. In a healthy relationship, you might feel nostalgia for those exciting early stages, but you can also accept reality and appreciate the security you now have with that person.

You can also habituate to experiences that aren't pleasurable. The first time I had to stick a needle into myself to administer a fertility drug, I was terrified. I spent hours leading up to the injections consumed by fear. Now, when it's time for the umpteenth needle, I still don't love it, but the intensity of my anticipation subsided with repeated exposure to the stimulus. Just as the response loses its intensity with repeated exposure, so does the anticipation that amps up (and exacerbates) that expected response.

Sometimes, when you've been suppressing an emotion or depriving yourself of an experience for a while, full permission can lead to a rebound effect. At first, it seems like the floodgates are opened and suddenly *all* you want are the foods you used to limit, and *all* you feel are the emotions you used to avoid or suppress. This rebound period is natural and temporary. If you continue to give yourself unconditional permission, you *will* eventually habituate.

My clients who were coming off opioids learned this the hard way. When they stopped chasing pleasure, for a while it seemed like the only sensation they could feel was pain. They felt chronically irritable, frustrated, or sad. After some time and stabilization, the full spectrum of emotions returned. They habituated to the unpleasant emotions they had previously numbed out, and as a result, experienced more emotional balance. Feelings of pleasure will never be as intense as the manufactured pleasure of a narcotic drug, but without the contrasting high highs of an artificial substance overwhelming the brain's receptors, those lows don't feel quite as low.

Seven-Day Habituation Challenge

To see habituation in action, try using this activity to take power away from a food that feels "bad" or indulgent to you. Choose a food you usually have rules or restrictions around. Eat this food every day for one week. For consistency, it's best to habituate to one food at a time, and use the same flavor and brand of the food every day.

Using the worksheet you can download at http://www.newharbinger .com/54063, write down the food you chose. Describe how you felt before, during, and after eating. Each day, rate how enjoyable it was, and whether your enjoyment changed from the previous day. Notice flavors, textures, and sensations as you eat. Notice how it feels in your body, and how much it takes to feel satisfied. Remember, you can eat as much as you want!

Repeat this activity for as many weeks as you need. Stop when you're truly tired of the chosen food, then repeat with a new formerly forbidden food. Throughout the process, notice any thoughts or feelings that arise with curiosity, not judgment.

Habituation can happen for anything you've previously put rules and restrictions around, from eating chips to crying to experiencing anger—with this exception: habituation does not apply to substances that create physical dependence, like tobacco, alcohol, or drugs. These substances should not be used for this activity. For naturally occurring experiences like food cravings or emotions, unconditional permission allows for those stimuli to become less overpowering. You can even habituate to the uncomfortable feeling that comes with letting people down!

My husband taught me this lesson early in our relationship. It turns out I married a fellow people-pleaser. Although our pleasing strategies look different, we both have trouble being honest when it might upset someone we love. For a while, I thought he had no opinions. Anytime I stated a preference, he went with it. His standard answer to "What do you want for dinner?" was always a breezy "Whatever you want." Then, every few months, seemingly out of nowhere, he'd lose his temper. Because he married a psychologist, he's frequently subjected to deep dives into our emotional and relational dynamics (he's a good sport). Soon it came to light that much of the time he wasn't really "fine with whatever," but he kept his opinion to himself to avoid disappointing me. Then, once dozens of moments of self-silencing piled up, he'd reach a breaking point and explode.

When he identified this pattern, I felt a kinship with him. After all, shutting down my needs to please others was my most practiced childhood pastime. But shutting down feelings doesn't make them disappear. While my style was to suppress until the emotional buildup sank me into a depressive black hole, his was to suppress until he exploded in a firework display of anger. (Perhaps it's no coincidence that when we did finally express, we each expressed in the way that was prescribed as most acceptable by our gender norms). As the saying goes, you can only sweep things under the rug for so long before they start coming out the other side.

Nowadays, we regularly disappoint each other. It's never fun to have to tell the other person that you don't want to do the thing they're suggesting, but in the end, we'd rather tolerate temporary disappointment than know the person we love is bottling their true feelings. Plus, when there's less suppression, there's also less explosion. If you're used to forcing things away, it can take time to warm up to the idea that your desires and emotions have unconditional permission to be there. We're trained to analyze and judge our instincts, but you don't have to automatically assume these experiences must be overpowered. When we make space for wants and needs, we can respond to them with greater clarity. By nonjudgmentally accepting them, we also take away their power.

If, like my husband, you've been habitually ignoring your true instincts and needs for a long time, you may struggle to know when you're suppressing them. You might start by exploring what you typically deny yourself—whether it's a particular food, emotion, or experience. If you're not sure what you're denying yourself, consider what you feel ashamed about. Sometimes, shame can highlight where you usually try to keep things buttoned up. Humans are messy and complicated. We cannot control our cravings and desires any more than we can control our need for oxygen. As you work on freeing yourself from overcontrol and giving yourself permission for the full spectrum of feelings, needs, and preferences, you might also find that burnout is a rarer experience.

The process begins with unconditional permission, but you also have to understand *what* you're giving yourself permission to feel or do. The remaining chapters in this section will help you discover ways to reopen the channels of communication between your mind and body, so you can tune in to your cravings and better recognize what you desire. Through a skill called interoceptive awareness, you'll become more familiar with your body's natural rhythms and signals, guiding you to meet its needs for hunger, satisfaction, comfort, emotional expression, and anything else it might be asking for.

Now that you hopefully see the value in making space for those experiences without judgment, you'll be open to learning more compassionate ways to respond to them. Remember that all of this work is designed to help you get off the hamster wheel you've been spinning on, exhausting yourself and going nowhere. When you know what you care about, recognize what you need, and care less about societal expectations, you can embrace a more authentic—and more fulfilling—version of your life.

CHAPTER 7

Tapping into Your Hunger

Tanya has been taking care of people for as long as she can remember, and she's really good at it. As the oldest, she was in charge of helping her younger siblings get ready for school each morning, and watching them after school while her parents were at work. As an adult, she lives with her long-term boyfriend and although they both work full time, she also takes on the brunt of the housework and packs his lunch most days. As her parents are aging, she also finds herself jumping in to care for them.

With all of her caretaking expertise, going into nursing was a natural decision. When she struggles, she prefers to keep it to herself. Although her friends are happy to support her through tough times, their empathy makes her uncomfortable. She'd much rather be the person doling out support than the one on the receiving end. When she started having episodes of anxiety and panic, the idea of going to therapy was pretty far outside her comfort zone. Eventually, her best friend convinced her to make an appointment.

Tanya's two goals for therapy were to manage stress better and to get her binge eating under control. Soon it became clear that for most of the day, attending to her needs wasn't a priority. Her mornings were often rushed, with a long commute to the hospital. She didn't eat breakfast, but never left home without her thirty-two-ounce thermos of coffee. At work, she'd grab a snack when there was time, but she didn't usually sit down to eat a full meal until getting home at night.

In the spirit of self-care, Tanya's therapist asked her to start eating breakfast. To help reduce anxiety, she was also encouraged to limit caffeine to one or two cups of coffee per day. After a few weeks of eating breakfast, she found herself surprisingly energized throughout the morning, but noticed that by the afternoon she got irritable. Her therapist explained how hunger cues can get quieter if they're ignored. Now that she was eating breakfast, the cues were coming back online. She realized her afternoon irritability was actually her body sending hunger signals, telling her it was time for lunch.

She also started to understand that fatigue was sometimes a sign of hunger. Previously, she thought she was just drained from work. She assumed she was fine eating very little all day, then having a big dinner. Now that she wasn't blunting her hunger cues with caffeine, her body was starting to tell her it needed food more consistently throughout the day. When she honored her hunger, she had more energy, emotional stability, and mental focus. Tanya discovered the power of attuning to her bodily signals through *interoceptive awareness*.

You're probably familiar with the five sensory systems (visual, auditory, olfactory, gustatory, and tactile), but did you know you actually have eight senses? Occupational therapists are well versed in the three lesser-known sensory systems, which include the *proprioceptive system* (attunement to your body's muscles to tell you about your position in space and which muscles are engaged), *vestibular system* (which tells you about any changes in your movement or balance), and *interoceptive system*. Your interoceptive system is responsible for perceiving and responding to signals within your body, such as hunger, thirst, heart rate, a full bladder, or pain sensations. Small children build interoceptive awareness through potty training, where they learn to use their brain to recognize the "gotta go" urge of a full bladder. Before that process, their bodies still excrete, but it's not under conscious control until they go through this attunement process.

Consider what's happening in your body right now, as you're reading this. Are you aware of how heavily or deeply you're breathing? How quickly your heart is beating? Whether any areas of your body are tight or in pain? If there was a change in your body's sensations (for instance, if you started getting hungry, thirsty, or having to use the bathroom), would you notice subtle shifts in intensity? Or would you not notice until your body was screaming at you?

Here are some ways you might practice developing interoceptive awareness in everyday life:

- Set a timer for thirty seconds and bring your attention to the involuntary processes in your body. Notice your breath going in and out, your eyes blinking, and your mouth swallowing at regular intervals.

- Do a brief body scan, either on your own or with guidance (try searching "guided body scan" on YouTube). Notice any areas of tightness, tension, or sensation as you move awareness from the crown of your head all the way through each body part, down to the tips of your toes.

- For one minute, place your hand over your heart and feel your heartbeat. Slowly remove your hand and see if you can still perceive your heartbeat, even without the tactile feedback of your hand on your chest.

- For one minute, feel your pulse (you can detect it by placing your index and middle fingers gently but firmly on your neck, just under the side of your jaw). Then remove your fingers and see if you can still perceive the pulsation without the tactile feedback.

- Next time you realize that you have the urge to use the restroom, pause and notice the sensation of a full bladder, and the sensation of emptying it.

Note: *If you have a trauma history, safety is crucial for building interoceptive awareness. As you try out these exercises, notice if you become overwhelmed or activated. If it's too challenging to connect to bodily sensations on your own, bring these activities to a therapist or trusted friend so you can practice them in a supportive environment.*

Interoception is necessary for maintaining well-being because it allows us to recognize physiological changes or imbalances, and take action to address them. Without that awareness, our needs can go ignored. Yet when we're consumed by toxic striving, we repeatedly tune out these signals, especially hunger signals, until there are consequences. Hunger cues are built into us from birth, as eating is a survival instinct basic to all living organisms. Even though infants can express when they're hungry, they have to fine-tune their interoception with practice. That fine-tuning might involve recognizing when you're hungry, how hungry you are, and how much food will satisfy that level of hunger for however long you want to be satisfied. Each of us feels hunger differently, but it usually involves a combination of mental and physical cues, whether a growling or gnawing sensation, watering mouth, irritability, difficulty focusing, or suddenly finding yourself thinking about food.

When you don't respond to hunger, the signals get more intense and unpleasant as your brain and body amp up the urgency to eat. You've probably experienced this at some point—you go from mildly hungry to hangry or ravenous. If after that intensity amps up, you *still* don't give your body food, the sensations then start to dull. This happens whether you deny yourself food intentionally by fasting or dieting, or whether you have no choice due to food insecurity. Your body doesn't know the difference between intentional and unintentional restriction. It just knows it's not getting a response to those hunger signals it's sending so frantically, so it figures there must be a famine. If there's a famine, your body doesn't want to waste precious energy sending you signals to find food, since there's clearly none available. Instead, it switches to conservation mode, slowing your metabolism and conserving energy until it's sufficiently fed.

It would be amazing if we all grew up with opportunities to listen to our bodies' messages. Sadly, this often isn't the case. For many chronic dieters, wellness junkies, and perfectionists, hunger and other bodily signals have been habitually ignored or misconstrued. Wellness and hustle cultures tell us to numb painful emotions, power through fatigue, overanalyze inner signals, and outsmart hunger and cravings. We learn to treat information from the body as inconvenient rather than important. We attempt to live from the neck up, preoccupied with the content of our minds and never dropping down into our bodies to gather information.

Even worse, we demonize not only our hunger but also our cravings for things beyond food. We learn to do what others want or expect, even if it doesn't align with our own desires. Instead of learning to meet our needs consistently and without judgment, we learn to ignore our bodies and make decisions based only on logic. We rarely practice attuning to instincts or honoring cravings, but we frequently practice numbing and disconnecting from ourselves.

Barriers to Interoceptive Awareness

- Trauma

- Grief

- Mood and anxiety disorders

- Eating disorders

- Lack of self-care practices

- Stress

- Illness

- Medications

- Substance use (including caffeine and nicotine)

- Conditions that affect how you take in sensory information

This is particularly true for people who experience trauma. Trauma can alter our neurological and psychological functioning. If you have been made to feel unsafe in your body or been violated through interpersonal violence, abuse, or assault, you may have learned to disconnect from your body as a form of self-protection. If you have been shamed for your weight or pressured into dieting from a young age, you may have learned not to trust your body a long time ago. There is also a high correlation between eating disorders and trauma (Brewerton 2007). If you have suffered from an eating disorder, with or without co-occurring trauma, you may have a warped sense of bodily signals, especially signals for hunger. Or if you have experienced food insecurity, it may not have mattered if you were hungry because you couldn't respond when there was no food available.

All of these experiences can create dissociation, disconnection, and distrust. To heal, it is vital to rebuild safety in your body. Understanding the nervous system can help you purposely cultivate that sense of inner safety. Through grounding practices like deep diaphragmatic breathing or guided relaxation exercises, you can communicate to your body that it is safe now. If you're healing from trauma, it is best to build these skills under the guidance of a trauma-informed psychotherapist or health care provider. It will also be helpful to have healing, supportive relationships with others in your community with whom you feel safe.

On a smaller scale, interoception is also affected by the stress response, also known as fight-or-flight. You can think of your nervous system as having two speeds—"fight or flight" and "rest and digest." You can't have both sides activated at the same time, so when the mobilization side is activated, the body is focused on getting through the stress. It doesn't signal you to seek food until it feels calm. Once you've come down from the intensity, you'll likely feel hungry again.

A similar effect can happen when you've just engaged in intense exercise; you may not feel hungry right afterward if your body is still activated. Drugs, alcohol, certain medications, caffeine, grief, depression, and anxiety can also affect appetite and hunger signals. Understanding how these factors impact hunger signals can help you remember that you still need to eat regularly, even without obvious cues. You can engage in *self-care eating*, using information from both your mind and body to determine whether to eat. When your appetite is not the best indicator of whether you need food, you can rely on your brain to tell you that it's still important to eat. Remember the binge-restrict cycle from chapter 6? If you go too long without eating, your body may drive you to binge once your hunger cues come back online. Eating regularly throughout the day also keeps blood sugar stable and helps you feel regulated, which can help ease mental and physical health symptoms.

Many people find that honoring their hunger becomes a gateway for honoring other unmet needs, including emotional needs. When Tanya turned her hunger signals back on, she opened the door to other important signals she had silenced. It all started with food. After a while, she was not only more aware of when she felt hungry, she was aware of what she was hungry for. She no longer felt stressed about cooking dinner or guilty when she ordered takeout. Her eating decisions were rooted in hunger, not rules.

Some nights, she ordered pizza because that was what her body genuinely wanted. Other nights, it was more appealing to her to have salmon and rice. She realized that if she listened to her body, it would tell her what it needed to feel satisfied.

Soon she was listening to her body when it gave her signals about her emotions. Emotions often show up as sensations in the body, such as a racing heart when excited, tightness in the chest when anxious, a pit in the stomach accompanying dread, feeling your blood "boiling" when you're angry, or buzzing with warmth when you feel joy. Building interoception allows for better emotional attunement and regulation. Tanya realized that when arguing with her boyfriend, she often felt an urge to make herself smaller. She recognized that in these interactions, she was feeling criticized and disrespected. Her therapist helped her learn to express herself more directly when feeling this way. The next time her body sent signals of being disrespected, Tanya told her boyfriend how she was feeling. Over time, her boyfriend made a conscious effort to speak more respectfully, and as a result, Tanya felt safer expressing herself. With more open communication, their relationship grew stronger. Developing interoceptive awareness helped Tanya realize many places in her life where she'd been self-silencing.

Reconnecting with Hunger Signals

Consider the following list of signals that people commonly experience when hungry. Place an X beside each cue you experience when mildly or moderately hungry. Place an ! beside each cue you experience when extremely hungry. If you experience signs of hunger that aren't listed here, write them in the blank spaces at the end.

Stomach and body cues:

____ Growling

____ Gurgling

____ Gnawing

____ Stomach pain or discomfort

____ Sense of stomach emptiness

____ Heartburn or acid reflux

____ Nausea

____ Burping

____ Salivating

____ Weird taste in your mouth

____ Dizziness

____ Other:

Mental and emotional cues:

____ Headaches

____ Anxiety or nervousness

____ Irritability, impatience, agitation

____ Increased difficulty making decisions

____ Fatigue or low energy

____ Restlessness

____ Losing focus, distractibility

____ Difficulty concentrating

____ Having more thoughts about food

____ Other:

Next, use the Hunger Log (available at http://www.newharbinger.com /54063) to track your hunger once per hour for a full day. At each checkpoint, you'll rate your levels of hunger and fullness, note any mental cues or physical sensations you felt, and write down what, if anything, you ate right before or after that checkpoint.

Note: *If you are in recovery from an eating disorder and it would be harmful to write down what you ate, please skip this portion of the exercise. You may also wish to skip this exercise entirely, and wait to complete it under the care and guidance of a therapist or dietitian who specializes in eating disorders.*

Keep in mind that when you're starting to pay attention to hunger cues, it's normal to be hyperconscious at first. With practice, you'll notice those cues without as much conscious effort. Remember that hunger doesn't always make sense. Sometimes you might be surprised how hungry you are so soon after eating a snack or meal. Other times, you might find that your hunger signals are pretty consistent or predictable. The important thing is to honor them when they arise, without judging or overanalyzing.

Neurodivergence and Interoception

If you are neurodivergent—for instance, if you have autism spectrum disorder (ASD) or attention-deficit/ hyperactivity disorder (ADHD), you may experience sensory processing differences, such as being more sensitive to light, sound, or various textures or smells (Kutscheidt et al. 2019; Miller et al. 2017). Considering that interoception is one of your sensory processing systems, it is not a surprise some neurodivergent people have trouble recognizing and responding to hunger, thirst, and other signals (Cobbaert and Rose 2023; Schmitt and Schoen 2022). Let's explore three common ways that neurodivergent people may struggle with interoception.

Underresponsivity: For someone with underresponsive interoception, inner signals can seem muted. This makes it hard to pick up on sensations of thirst (which can lead to dehydration), and hunger (which may cause them to miss meals, have blood sugar imbalances, or even develop an eating disorder), and pain signals (which may lead to missing signs of illness or injury until the condition becomes more serious or threatening). Underresponders may also struggle to recognize when they're full. In children, underresponsivity may make potty training difficult. Underresponsive individuals might also struggle to pick up on emotions until they become overpowering, leading to unintentional outbursts or tantrums.

These tips can help: (1) if you typically forget to eat, drink water, or use the bathroom, setting notifications on your phone or alarms to go off at specific times can help you remember to attend to basic needs without a physical signal; (2) a dietitian can help you determine appropriate energy needs for your body and activity level, so that you can ensure you're eating enough on a regular basis; or (3) you can also create a schedule for regular mealtimes and bedtimes, and make regular appointments for preventative health care, to help ensure that you're attending to your body's needs even without loud inner signals.

Overresponsivity: People who are overresponsive may feel like their sensory signals are heightened and intense (Istvan, Nevill, and Mazurek 2020; Lane, Reynolds, and Thacker 2010). Rather than getting progressively hungrier until they are ready for a meal, they may find the slightest hunger signal unbearable. Rather than feeling a slowly developing urge to urinate, they might perceive any amount of urine in the bladder as a sign to immediately use the bathroom. Someone who is overresponsive may feel that even the slightest pain or discomfort is a reason to seek medical attention. They might be hypersensitive to the slightest shift in mood or emotional state, making them feel dysregulated in the presence of stimuli that might not seem overwhelming to others. As a result, "overresponsiveness can make an individual avoidant of activities, different textures [and] foods, or input for fear of the heightened response they experience" (E. Wickenkamp, OTR/L, personal communication, January 30, 2024).

These tips can help: (1) if you tend to overrespond, you might benefit from more frequent, smaller meals and snacks throughout the day, and find it soothing to know when the next meal or break is coming; and (2) overresponders sometimes find stimming behaviors soothing, and may turn to eating for added stimulation. While there is nothing wrong with eating for stimulation, it can help to have a variety of tools, beyond food, for providing stimulation throughout the day. You might try going for walks, playing with a fidget toy, wrapping yourself tightly in a blanket, bouncing on a small trampoline, or banging on a drum.

Discrimination difficulties: Those with discrimination difficulties have trouble discerning what their bodily signals are telling them. They might be unclear whether the sensation they're feeling is a sign of hunger, thirst, sickness, or anxiety. It can also be challenging to recognize which emotions they're feeling, making it hard to self-regulate. While the sensations that accompany emotions can often feel similar for everyone (for example, most people have a racing heart when they feel nervous), someone with discrimination difficulties might not know whether their heart is racing because of anxiety, excitement, or something else. Physical sensations often feel disorganized and confusing, and they might respond with panic or make wild guesses about what their body needs.

These tips can help: (1) you may benefit from a schedule of regular breaks and mealtimes, and having ready-to-eat snacks on hand; (2) when you're unsure whether you're hungry, you can experiment with a bite or small snack, and notice if it has an impact on how you feel; (3) if you don't get more stereotypical signs like a headache or growling stomach, you may look for changes in mood or behavior to signal that you're hungry; or (4) a helpful rule of thumb is to plan to eat something, even something small, every three hours during the day, to keep your blood sugar steady.

Knowledge Is Power

You can learn to support yourself, even if your signals look different from someone else's. An occupational therapist who specializes in sensory processing difficulties can help you figure out what works best for you. If you don't have access to an OT, you can search for resources online, using the term "interoception."

You probably wouldn't think it was the best idea to put on a blindfold before heading down a busy street, or wear noise-canceling headphones at your favorite concert. Yet in wellness and hustle cultures, we are taught to cut ourselves off from important sensory information. If we're hungry, we question whether it's acceptable to eat. When we're tired, we just pour another cup of coffee, trying to eke out a bit more work. Reopening the lines of communication between your mind and your body can lead to a greater sense of stability in your everyday life. You don't have to wait for your body to get to a place of extreme discomfort before responding.

Recognizing unmet needs allows you to address them. The other half of that equation is being able to recognize when you've had enough—when you're satisfied. Sadly, just as many of us are taught to fear, ignore, or distort our hunger signals, we also learn to disconnect from signals of pleasure, fullness, or satisfaction. In a culture that glorifies discipline and deprivation, fullness can feel uncomfortable or laced with shame, as if we are bad for honoring cravings. Aversion to fullness can go hand in hand with a fear of gaining weight, fueled by the pressure to take up as little space as possible. Alternatively, some people are so sensitive to sensations of hunger or so overwhelmed by having an unmet need that they swing to the other extreme. For them, fullness can feel like a safety net that is never quite sturdy enough.

In chapter 8, you'll explore fullness, and what it means to you. Just as honoring hunger can serve as a gateway into recognizing hunger for other things you need, crave, or desire, so can your experience of physical fullness serve as a gateway. Learning to honor signals of fullness can also help you honor whatever else makes you feel soothed and satisfied in everyday life. Despite what you may have been taught, you deserve to experience satisfaction. Once you've untangled from negative associations with pleasure and fullness, you can start opening up to what fulfills you physically, mentally, emotionally, and spiritually.

CHAPTER 8

Embracing Fullness and Satisfaction

Allie sat alone at her cousin's wedding reception, watching a group of relatives dance wildly to "YMCA." After a few trips to the dessert buffet, she was uncomfortably full. She felt her Spanx digging into her stomach and cursed herself for wearing such a form-fitting dress. She'd avoided carbs all week to prepare for this event. When the dessert came out, she decided to reward herself with an iced sugar cookie, but one cookie soon became eight. Now, as her loved ones celebrated, she sat nursing a stomachache and planning what she'd eat this week to get back on track.

The feeling of fullness was complicated for Allie. Growing up, she was fortunate to always know where her next meal would come from, but under her mom's watchful eye, she still couldn't trust she'd get enough. If she reached for seconds, her mom would ask, "Are you sure you want more?" It seemed like she was supposed to stop eating *before* she got full, so she learned to associate being full with overdoing it. She struggled to find a comfortable place where she had eaten enough to be satisfied and wasn't left wanting more. She would closely monitor her food at most meals, but if her guard was down after having a few drinks, or if she was eating something she usually restricted, she had trouble stopping herself. Then, when she got very full, the sensations felt unbearable. To her, that level of fullness meant she had eaten too much, and she complained to her friends that she felt fat.

Hunger is one of our most basic survival needs. It makes sense then that fullness is a precursor to being able to think clearly and feel stable. If you don't honor hunger, you'll likely become preoccupied with food. As we explored in the last chapter, this is one important way that our bodies drive us to do what we need to survive. Once we are safe and fed, the stress response of fight-or-flight deactivates and allows us to turn our attention to other pursuits. Yet our social conditioning can teach us to distort or disregard this basic need. The ability to attune to fullness becomes clouded, and we struggle to recognize it as a positive signal. Wellness culture tells us to hyperfixate on portion sizes and be careful not to eat too much, which can lead us to stop before we've truly had enough. If we ever eat beyond that place, it seems like we've gone overboard or lost control. Many people question their hunger or try to outsmart it. You might have learned that if you think you're hungry, you're probably just thirsty or tired, so you should try drinking water or taking a walk.

In other situations, fullness is fraught with a different meaning. Unfortunately, for many people, the opportunity for fullness isn't a given. If you have experienced trauma or food insecurity, it's possible that fullness feels elusive or foreign. Some people may experience fullness as a rarity, a special treat that must be clung to or stored up for later. Instead of being afraid of becoming too full, you might be afraid of not being full enough. If you're no longer experiencing food insecurity, having an abundance of food in your home may help soothe that part of you. Reassuring your body that there *is* enough food can help it relax, trusting that it won't be deprived again.

Note: *If you're currently experiencing food insecurity, getting consistent food is a top priority. If you live in the United States, check out feedingamerica.org to locate your nearest food bank.*

Fullness can also be tied to emotional coping. Since food is often our earliest form of comfort, many people learn to use it to soothe themselves even when they're not hungry. This is not something to demonize. If you turn to food for comfort, and it helps you, that's great! You have a reliable tool for comforting yourself. However, it's usually helpful to have more than one tool in your toolkit. You don't want food to be your *only* option for comfort, in case it's ever unavailable or ineffective. If you can recognize food as one of many options for comfort, you can also get curious about other things that might comfort you, such as cuddling a pet or loved one, wrapping in a cozy blanket, taking a warm shower or bath, or watching your favorite movie. The more options you have for comfort, the more precise you can be in choosing the tool that's going to help you the most in a given situation.

What if you get too full? Several factors make it harder to notice when you've reached comfortable fullness:

When you're eating food laced with rules. When you eat something you previously had (or currently have) rules about, you might struggle to notice fullness signals. We tend to feel out of control around whichever foods we've tried hardest to control. Giving yourself unconditional permission to eat as much of that food as you'd like, as often as you'd like, will help that food become more neutral over time.

When you're extremely hungry. We tend to eat more, eat faster, and be less aware of fullness signals when extremely we're hungry than when we're only mildly or moderately hungry. Paying attention to hunger signals and responding to them before they reach that level of extreme intensity can help you slow down and notice how your body is responding to the food.

When you're eating while distracted. If you're watching television, working, or scrolling your phone while eating, it's easy to lose touch with your body signals. While it's natural and sometimes even practical to eat while doing other things, you can still bring awareness to your body to notice when you've reached comfortable fullness. Intuitive eating cofounder Evelyn Tribole (2020) recommends pausing at your first bite, a "middle" bite, and one of your last bites to notice how you're feeling and recognize body signals, even if you're distracted for the other parts of the meal.

Even if you're generally attuned to your signals, you might still end up uncomfortably full sometimes. It happens! If you get to that place, don't panic. While it may be unpleasant, it's also temporary. No matter how full you are, your body will eventually digest the food and the discomfort will subside. You may feel urges to compensate for eating past the point your body needed. If you can instead sit with the sensations and offer yourself compassion, you'll come out of this temporary feeling in a stronger headspace.

Try owning the mantra "Whoops, I got a little too full!" No big deal. If you make it into something to berate yourself over, you'll only increase your anxiety the next time you eat. Instead, trust that your body will tell you when it's hungry again, and you'll honor that hunger when it shows up. You can also get curious about what might have made it hard to recognize when you were comfortably full in that scenario. Were you extremely hungry? Commit to noticing milder hunger signals and honoring them sooner next time. Were you distracted? Commit to being a bit more present next time, then forgive yourself and move on. Accidentally eating more than your body wanted is not a crime.

In graduate school, I took a course on family therapy. We watched a video where the therapist worked with a family whose only daughter, at the time a young adult, was suffering from severe anorexia. The therapist explored the family's history and dynamics, and offered an interesting hypothesis about the girl's symptoms. He wondered whether the family was inadvertently encouraging the girl to stay small, not just physically but developmentally. It seemed her parents and siblings unconsciously wanted her to remain childlike, to remain their little girl instead of letting her grow and become a self-sufficient adult.

When someone is malnourished, as is often the case with anorexia nervosa, their body will regress. They might stop getting their period and lose their sex drive. They might grow a fine layer of hair, called lanugo, similar to what appears on a baby in utero. These are biological mechanisms designed to protect a starving body. From a psychological perspective, it's interesting to consider how deprivation sends someone back to a more childlike, fragile, and dependent state. Anorexia and other eating disorders have a variety of causes and contributing factors. They do not always stem from a family dynamic that promotes immaturity or regression. However, examples like this illustrate just how insidious the pressure to stay small can be for so many people, particularly women and femmes.

The belief that it's good to be small, thin, toned, shredded, or whatever language your mind latches onto, is ingrained even for people who do not struggle with an eating disorder. Beliefs about body size are conditioned into us in the same ways that other beliefs are instilled—through our families, communities, media messaging, cultures, and society at large. Explicitly and implicitly, we absorb ideas about what it means to take up space, literally and figuratively.

Even if you don't subscribe on a conscious level to the idea that thinness is superior to fatness, you probably hold some beliefs about what size you should be. There is stigma associated with being in a larger body, and thus, it is understandable that you might be fearful of gaining weight. Likewise, if you live in a body that's been discriminated against for size, it's understandable if you want to lose weight. That's the damage of a fatphobic society. Just because it's the way things are doesn't mean it's okay. Consider the beliefs you identified at the beginning of this book regarding body size and what your body "should" be like. When you think of your biases about body size, how do they square up with your personal values?

We absorb ideas not only about what it means to take up physical space but also to take up space through our personalities and social roles. We learn what it means to be quiet versus loud, to have strong opinions versus going with the flow. We learn what it means about us if we seek attention or feel comfortable in the spotlight. We're supposed to be conservative, but not prudish. Sexually expressive, but not slutty. Confident, but not cocky. Smart, but not intimidating. Patriarchal expectations for women and femmes are typically unachievable. It's no wonder so many people struggle to know what it feels like to be at ease, comfortable, or satisfied.

I remember several years ago when the term "manspreading" came into the vernacular. The local news did a puff piece showing footage of headless white men on public transportation, sitting with their legs spread across several seats, their bags beside them, seemingly oblivious to the disproportionate space they took up as other passengers crowded to the edge of the car. Since then, mansplaining has also entered the cultural chat. We're putting words to concepts that have long been normalized in society, where men (particularly white men) are automatically entitled to more space and more airtime than everyone else, for no other reason than the fact that they are white men. They receive the message that it's not only acceptable to be loud and loom large, but it's actually the right thing for them to do. Meanwhile, to uphold this system, the rest of us have to do our part to stay out of the way. We're taught that it's our job to take up less space, to make ourselves small and unobtrusive and pleasing.

I've often wondered who benefits from a world where women and femmes are fearful of taking up space. Sure, technically, men and others with privilege benefit, because when everyone else cooperates with staying small, we uphold the system that keeps those with privilege in positions of power. But do they really benefit in the end? That power keeps people comfortable, but it also keeps them stagnant.

When everything is designed to keep you comfortable at all costs, you miss out on having true, meaningful, authentic, life-enriching interactions. When people are tiptoeing around you, focused on pleasing or accommodating you, those interactions don't foster growth or connection. We grow by being pushed outside our comfort zones, receiving feedback, thinking critically, and getting honest with ourselves. We grow by facing challenges and adversity. We grow by engaging with people who are different from us, and who experience the world through a different lens. Although the patriarchy is most harmful to those with the least social privilege, at the end of the day, the system hurts all of us. It keeps us catering to a collectively unfulfilling status quo instead of expressing our full potential as unique human beings.

Remember that you're part of the system, and by doing the inside job of unlearning your biases and challenging beliefs about how you should be, you can help chip away at these harmful cultural assumptions. Maybe you've absorbed the message that taking up space is wrong, but do you believe this to be true, deep down? Remind yourself of your values and priorities as you begin to think about fullness, satisfaction, and taking up space. In a culture that promotes self-deprivation, it can be radical to prioritize pleasure. If you've been conditioned to believe you must stay small, it might be hard to imagine a life where you get to do things simply because they enrich your life.

Pleasure can come in a variety of forms. I find pleasure when I stare at the flickering flame of my favorite candle, place the last piece of a jigsaw puzzle, or cut into the runny yolk of a perfectly poached egg. Pleasure might come with the release of a deep tissue massage, an orgasm, or a really amazing chocolate truffle. Do any of these experiences dramatically change someone or solve any big problems? Probably not, but they make life fuller! Without those random bits of pleasure, your life would probably look the same from the outside, but from the inside, it would feel a little emptier. Your sources of pleasure are well worth discovering. You might start with food, and tune in to what you're craving by asking yourself what appeals to you. Then, you can move into exploring other sources of pleasure and satisfaction in your life, both big and small.

Discovering Pleasure, Part 1: What Am I Craving?

Learning to recognize what you're craving can bring you closer to finding satisfaction with food. Next time you're hungry, try to catch your hunger signals at a mild or moderate level of intensity, and use this this exercise. Check all that apply, and then consider some options that fit what you're seeking.

Temperature:

☐ Hot

☐ Warm

☐ Room temperature

☐ Cold

☐ Combination of: _____

☐ Other: _____

Taste:

☐ Savory   ☐ Sugary

☐ Sweet   ☐ Salty

☐ Sour   ☐ Rich

☐ Tart   ☐ Nutty

☐ Umami   ☐ Tangy

☐ Earthy   ☐ Spicy

☐ Buttery   ☐ Fruity

☐ Combination of: _____

☐ Other: _____

Texture:

- ☐ Crunchy
- ☐ Crispy
- ☐ Smooth
- ☐ Soft
- ☐ Firm

- ☐ Creamy
- ☐ Liquidy
- ☐ Hearty
- ☐ Thick
- ☐ Chewy

- ☐ Melty
- ☐ Oily
- ☐ Dry
- ☐ Grainy
- ☐ Light and airy

- ☐ Combination of: _____
- ☐ Other: _____

Visual appeal:

- ☐ Colorful and diverse
- ☐ Stacked/ piled on a plate
- ☐ Several little dishes

- ☐ Together in a bowl
- ☐ Straight out of the container
- ☐ Topped, garnished, or drizzled

- ☐ Combination of: _____
- ☐ Other: _____

Aromas:

- ☐ Sweet (sugar, vanilla, cinnamon)
- ☐ Zesty (lemon, citrus, vinegar)
- ☐ Savory (garlic, butter, onion)

- ☐ Smokey (grilled, charred, mesquite)
- ☐ Fresh (bright, fruity, juicy)
- ☐ Spicy (pepper, wasabi, horseradish)

- ☐ Combination of: _____
- ☐ Other: _____

Eating experience:

- ☐ Fork and knife
- ☐ Spoon
- ☐ Chopsticks
- ☐ Finger food
- ☐ Hand-held
- ☐ Bite into, or cut up
- ☐ Messy, saucy, drippy
- ☐ Combination of: _____
- ☐ Other: _____

- ☐ Crumbly
- ☐ Just a nibble
- ☐ Snack
- ☐ Light meal
- ☐ Meal with staying power
- ☐ Big feast

Sometimes there are a few options that match your cravings. For example, if you crave sweet, creamy, and cold, you might like a cup of frozen yogurt, a milkshake, or a bowl of pudding. If you're craving savory, melty, and warm, you might enjoy grilled cheese, pizza, or a quesadilla. Other times, you want one specific food, and it's the only one that will do.

With practice, you'll get better at noticing what you desire without having to go through this whole exercise. It's not always realistic to have the exact food you want; I don't have the opportunity to eat filet mignon or fresh pasta with truffles as often as I wish! Still, you can use your cravings to get closer to the general vicinity of what appeals to you, and find satisfaction in the process. You can also consider how you wish to feel after eating. If certain foods make you feel energized and others make you sleepy, use this knowledge to honor what you need in a given situation both physically and emotionally.

There's a popular saying in eating disorder recovery communities: "You can't have a full life without a full stomach." Having a front-row seat to so many people's recovery processes, I can confirm that this is the case. My favorite part of helping clients recover is getting to discover who they actually are, once they begin breaking free from the all-consuming preoccupation with food, or with perfection. Sometimes, a client doesn't even know what they're interested in because their striving efforts have been their main focus for so long. Together, we discover that they actually love traveling, reading science fiction, or gardening. They're obsessed with the British royal family, or *Game of Thrones*, or vintage cars. They take an improv class, adopt a child, or go back to school to become a guidance counselor. They learn about their sexuality. They discover parts of themselves that make them feel more alive, more whole.

A lifetime of heavy participation in wellness and hustle cultures can have toxic effects on you. It's often not until you stop striving that you realize just how much energy you'd been devoting to those efforts.

Discovering Pleasure, Part 2: What Fills Me Up?

As comfortable fullness and satisfaction with food become more familiar, you can start opening up to other things that bring you a sense of fullness and satisfaction beyond food. Consider these questions, and jot down your reflections in your journal.

When you think of the word "pleasure," what comes to your mind? Is the general vibe positive, negative, or neutral?

What are some moments in the last few days that brought you pleasure or were satisfying to you? Describe at least one moment in great detail.

Where were you?

What was happening?

Describe the full sensory experience: sights, sounds, smells, textures, flavors, shapes, colors, and anything else that made it enjoyable for you.

When you pay attention, you might discover a million little things that light you up, a mosaic of fulfilling moments and activities that bring you bits of satisfaction. A delicious meal, singing along to a catchy new song on the radio, putting on your favorite cozy sweatshirt, or sharing a funny meme can all fill you up on any given day. Start a list in your journal, and commit to documenting one small moment of pleasure each day.

Satisfaction and pleasure often depend on context. Sometimes, you find something fulfilling because of its novelty or variety. Maybe your satisfaction comes from doing something you've been craving or looking forward to for a while. Maybe you're satisfied by an element of surprise, when something turns out different than what you expected. Maybe you're satisfied because you were present with all of the sensory elements of the experience—you really relished it and let yourself enjoy it. There's no universal formula for a satisfying experience, and what satisfies you one day may not hit the spot another day. If you tune in and pay attention though, you can figure out what might do it for you in any given moment.

In wellness and hustle cultures, there's not a lot of space to relish fulfilling experiences. Satisfaction is hypothetical. It's held up as the reward for achieving everything on your to-do list, but you're never actually encouraged to relish it. According to hustle culture, if you were to truly seek pleasure, you'd be hedonistic, indulgent, or frivolous. But pleasure does not have to come at the expense of our other priorities. In fact, making room for pleasure in your life can fill your tank, allowing you more energy to put toward whatever else is important to you.

You're on this planet for only a limited amount of time. If you have a clear sense of your values, you likely know what type of life you want to lead while you're here. Where does enjoyment or pleasure factor into your life's goals? Maybe you want to leave this world better off than you found it, or create a legacy for generations to come. Maybe you care about creating a certain type of environment for your family or loved ones, or making your mark on your professional field. These are wonderful pursuits, and they don't have to come at the expense of satisfaction. Humans are capable of caring about multiple things at once! Every day, no matter how busy you are, you encounter opportunities to experience satisfaction. Commit to doing one thing today for no other reason than because it fills you up.

When you consider your life through the lens of fullness and satisfaction, you can make space for any number of things that matter to you. Instead of having to single-mindedly fixate on being productive, you can explore what it means to be a whole person, with a full life that includes what mindfulness teacher Dr. Jon Kabat-Zinn (2013) often refers to as "the full catastrophe." You can make space for the ups and downs, laughter and tears, joy and pain, wins and losses that make life meaningful. It might seem counterintuitive to think about pain and unpleasant experiences as part of a fulfilling and rewarding life, but they are actually crucial pieces of the puzzle. We cannot know happiness without sadness. If there is no context for an emotion, it has no shape.

In the next chapter, we will explore how your emotional world can enhance your life and deepen the meaning you find in each day. Emotions—even the ones you dislike the most—aren't so intolerable once you know how to interpret them and move through them effectively. It's all about learning to speak their language and open yourself up to the messages they bring.

CHAPTER 9

Your Emotions Carry Messages

When I think back to elementary school, a single refrain jumps out in my mind: "We never have to worry about Paula!" This line was uttered by my parents, teachers, babysitters, and basically every adult who'd been tasked with the apparently very easy job of caring for me. That sentence made me glow with pride. It became my private mission to get people to repeat it as often as possible. *Nobody had to worry about me!* I was so well-behaved, so quiet, so agreeable. Everyone knew I would always follow the rules, and I didn't need too much attention or take up too many resources. I was an easy child, and it was clear that being easy was what was desired of me.

Adults seemed to conflate having needs with being needy, which I read as code for less lovable. I saw their looks of exasperation whenever another child threw a tantrum, and knew that if they ever looked that way at me, I would simply die of shame. Not having to worry about me was a compliment, which meant that if I required care, it was a negative thing. Meanwhile, below the surface I was desperate to be soothed and nurtured. Even a responsible, agreeable child has needs, but I had swallowed the belief that having needs was unacceptable. I deeply craved attention, but I had no idea how to get it without losing my status as "easy." So I became an expert in pretending my needs didn't exist, and drowned in guilt anytime the mask slipped.

As a teen and young adult, I suppressed my emotions until they forced their way out through panic attacks and bouts of depression. I developed an on-and-off eating disorder. Instead of communicating directly when I was hurting, I acted out through binge drinking and obsessive exercising. Perhaps on a subconscious level, I hoped someone would notice and care. Yet like many people, I believed that denial of my feelings and desires was the only way to get through life. I found partners who confirmed this belief, who were drawn to me because they wanted someone low maintenance. Eventually they would get fed up when, spoiler alert, I would show signs of having preferences. By adulthood, I had become an expert in self-silencing—the process of repeatedly suppressing thoughts, feelings, or needs and holding back from expressing them to others.

Self-silencing is usually an attempt to preserve a relationship, protect yourself, or please and placate others. It often develops as a survival strategy. You learn that it's best for your physical and/or emotional well-being to deny what you feel and appease the world around you. These tendencies can start in childhood or adolescence, and are most common for those socialized as female. While self-silencing might protect you from rejection or discomfort in the short run, over time it can make you sicker. Studies show that self-silencing behaviors are correlated with higher rates of depression, anxiety, body dissatisfaction, disordered eating, and chronic illness (Jack and Dill 1992; Maji and Dixit 2019; Shouse and Nilsson 2011).

If you've ever felt the relief of venting, or crying tears you've been holding back, picture the toxic effect of doing the opposite and holding it in, over and over. It's not just about the harm of suppressing emotions, it's also about the harm of not getting the validation and soothing that comes from another person receiving your emotions with warmth. We all not only deserve but deep down *need* this opportunity to be witnessed. This is one of the most powerful elements of psychotherapy—it's a place where you're completely free to express your emotions and have them met with unconditional acceptance. My own foray into therapy taught me this. Being witnessed in such a healing way was so moving that it led me to change my career path and become a psychologist myself!

Understanding Your Emotional World

If you relate to the experience of self-silencing, take a moment to reflect on your early emotional education. These questions can help you understand how you came to hide or avoid certain emotions. Feel free to jot down takeaways in your journal.

Which emotions were met with positivity or warmth by your parents or caregivers? (If it was different for each parent, indicate that too).

Which emotions were expressed the most freely in your home growing up?

Were the rules different for different family members? For example, was it acceptable for one person to express anger or sadness, but other family members weren't allowed to show these feelings?

How did the adults in your life respond when you felt happy? Sad? Angry? When you felt things were unfair?

When you were in a good mood, what was the response?

When you were cranky or in a bad mood, what was the response?

How did you ask for attention or care when you were craving it? How did the people in your life respond to those requests?

In your closest friendships of childhood, which emotions did you feel safe to express?

In romantic relationships or dating, do you try to control the other person's perception of your emotions? How do you want them to perceive you?

Why is this perception important to you?

You may attempt to control your emotions not only to accommodate others but also because you just don't like them. In ACT, we call efforts to try to control our inner worlds *experiential avoidance* and *experiential control*. We use experiential avoidance when we try to prevent or get rid of unwanted thoughts, feelings, or sensations, and we use experiential control when we try to cling to or prolong pleasant thoughts, feelings, and sensations. Our desire to control what we think and feel can even motivate us to act in ways that end up hurting ourselves or others.

For example, imagine your boss asks you to stay late to finish a task, and when you comply, he showers you with praise. That gives you a warm, pleasant feeling. Before you know it, you're chasing that warm glow at all costs, taking on extra work and behaving like a doormat. Or imagine that your partner breaks up with you unexpectedly. You feel the painful sting of rejection, decide you never want to feel that sting again, and develop a pattern of pulling away from potential partners at the first sign of intimacy.

The more you try to control what you feel, the more elusive your desired feelings become, *and* the more you suffer consequences. You end up focusing so much on feeling good or not feeling bad that you miss out on opportunities that make life worthwhile, like standing up for what you believe in, maintaining work/life balance, or fostering connections with loved ones. Or, if you're like me, you become so afraid of being seen as "too much" that you silence yourself at any indication that someone is annoyed or upset with you. These efforts can become a full-time job, consuming all of your energy and leaving you too depleted to pursue the things that feel meaningful to you.

This is why it's so freeing to make peace with your emotions—especially the painful ones. Whether you like it or not, being alive involves some degree of pain that is unavoidable. You fall and break your arm, and it hurts. You get dumped, and it hurts. A loved one passes away, and it hurts. There's no way for these things to not hurt. In that regard, pain is a natural, unavoidable experience that comes with being human.

We can unintentionally make that natural pain worse for ourselves through suffering. We create suffering by fighting against our pain, getting caught up in thoughts about how it's not fair, looking for someone or something to blame, or beating ourselves up for experiencing pain. We create suffering by stewing over feelings of anger, resentment, frustration, impatience, or hopelessness. We create suffering by searching for ways to "solve" pain through avoidance or control efforts: numbing out through drinking, drugs, binge eating, or purging; seeking control through restricting, overexercising, ignoring or distorting reality, or any number of other strategies that may temporarily distract or numb us, but ultimately lead to greater suffering.

Recall from chapter 6 that the antidote to this inner struggle is to give yourself unconditional permission to feel. Practicing acceptance of unwanted emotions will free you from the fight against them. Acceptance is tricky because many people interpret it to mean you have to like what you're feeling. But accepting the feeling of fear that arises in your body when you get up to give a presentation doesn't mean you like that feeling or that you want it to be there. It just means you're allowing it to exist. The alternative would be to get upset about the fact that you're feeling that way (which may make the feeling more intense), or to opt out of speaking opportunities to avoid the fear (which would mean giving up something meaningful).

Accepting what you cannot control is an intelligent choice, because it frees up your energy and resources to go toward the things you can control. The pain and difficulties of everyday life won't disappear, but you'll have a different (and likely less exhausting) relationship with life's hardships. You'll be better equipped to act in ways that match your values, so that you can feel proud of yourself looking back on your day, even if you went through some difficult feelings. In fact, while this isn't the goal of acceptance, it can also take the intensity away from those tough emotions. You might still feel sad, scared, lonely, or helpless sometimes, but those same feelings might be just a smidge less bothersome, because you're not fighting them, and because you know they're temporary. As I often remind my clients, feelings don't need fixing; they just need time.

Moving Through Tough Emotions

Next time you're having an intense emotion, try using this activity to approach it with acceptance and curiosity; you can follow along here or download the steps at http://www.newharbinger.com/54063.

Scan your body from head to toe. Notice any areas of sensation, and describe them. Which parts of your body have sensation? What is the sensation like—is it big, small, heavy, light, tight, loose, sharp, stabbing, throbbing, aching, tingling, numb, hot, cold? Are there edges to the sensation? Is there a shape, color, image, noise, texture, or flavor?

Do the sensations change when you start to describe them? Do they move around to other parts of your body, become more intense or less intense, or go away?

Now, try to self-regulate by using one of these strategies:

- Take five or six slow, deep breaths. Inhale deeply and fill your belly. Then exhale slowly and steadily.

- Wiggle your toes. Press your feet into the ground below you. Straighten your spine, and roll your shoulders a few times.

- Find a scented candle and inhale, noticing the smell.

- Put on scented lotion or dab essential oils on your wrists, and notice the scent.

- Hold an ice cube and feel the sensation of coldness in your hand.

- Pick a color, then scan your surroundings and notice everything around you that contains that color.

- Splash water on your face, then dab it dry with a towel.

Which regulation strategy did you try? What happened to the emotions as you used that strategy?

Remember, your goal is not to make the emotions or sensations go away. They will eventually go away on their own. Your job is just to pay attention and notice what's happening, and whether these strategies make it a bit easier to tolerate the emotion while it's happening.

Don't Kill the Messenger

Most of us don't receive the best emotional education growing up. By the time we reach adulthood, we might have some emotional awareness, but it often needs to be fine-tuned. It's like going from basic conversational skills in a foreign language to becoming fluent. In fact, you can think of emotions as a sort of language, communicating various messages to you. Being able to discern what you're feeling, and what might be underneath those feelings, is incredibly useful.

I first learned this idea of treating inner signals as messengers from mindfulness teacher Dr. Jon Kabat-Zinn. His approach, mindfulness-based stress reduction (MBSR), involves helping people change their relationship with pain by accepting it. MBSR helps the pain feel less intense and upsetting, even if the pain itself doesn't go away. In *Full Catastrophe Living* (2013), Dr. Kabat-Zinn explains that pain, and your feelings about it, are often bringing you messages. He writes, "In the old days, if a king didn't like the message he was given, he would sometimes have the messenger killed. This is tantamount to suppressing your symptoms or your feelings because they are unwanted." When you ignore or deny your pain, you may think you're moving toward relief. However, the message that the pain was trying to bring to you doesn't disappear. Killing the messenger it only makes the message more garbled and harder to understand.

Meanwhile, if you pay attention without judgment, you can recognize the message. Physical pain often has clear messages: the pain of a sprained ankle reminds you not to bear weight on it while it heals. The discomfort of a head cold reminds you to drink fluids and get extra rest while your body fights the illness. Emotional signals can be tougher to interpret. What does the pain of heartbreak communicate? Perhaps its message is in what that relationship meant to you, or how deeply you want to love another person in the future. The pain of grief can bring you the message of how much you miss the person who is gone, and remind you not to take loved ones for granted. The pain of feeling dismissed by a friend can bring you the message that some boundary setting is in order.

Similarly, pleasant and enjoyable emotions can also bring useful information. Feelings of love can help bond you to your partner or child and remind you to invest in your attachment to them. Feeling moved as you watch a happy couple share their wedding vows, or feeling happiness as your new puppy licks your face can keep you grounded in the present, reminding you to witness all of life's richness. When you make space for the full spectrum of your emotions without trying to control them, you can open up to the valuable sources of information they bring.

There are certainly times when an emotion can bring with it a distorted message. Thanks to conditioning, our emotional reactions aren't always pure indications of something that matters to us. Guilt is one of these often distorted emotions that many toxic strivers struggle to interpret. If you were taught by your family, community, or society that you *should* be a certain way, you might feel guilty when you deviate from that standard. Because I was conditioned to accommodate others even when it hurt me, I didn't learn to communicate assertively until adulthood. As a result, I still experience guilt as an immediate internal response to asserting myself. When I tell someone not to yell at me, or decline an invitation because I'm socially tapped out, I often feel a pang of guilt, as if I did something wrong. Deep down I know I'm allowed to protect my well-being, but I still have remnants of that old fear that if I don't succumb to others' wishes, I'll be deemed unlovable.

This guilt is different from the guilt that indicates you've behaved in a way that doesn't align with your values. As someone who values kindness, I feel guilty when I participate in gossip. In that scenario, guilt is actually an important messenger, showing up to discourage me from future gossipy behavior.

So how can you tell whether guilt—or any other emotion—is delivering an important message, or whether it's just a reflection of your conditioning? You may have to do some light detective work. Consider the context in which the guilt is showing up, and then reflect on the values you identified in chapter 5. If you were behaving in a way that aligned with the type of person you wish to be, and you still felt guilty, perhaps that guilt reflects your conditioning. If this is the case, it can be helpful to name what's going on (*I'm feeling guilty because I chose not to succumb to the pressures and expectations I'm facing*) and then offer yourself some compassion (*Everyone feels this way sometimes! I'm only human, and humans feel icky sometimes. I know this hard feeling will pass eventually, and I will survive it.*). With practice, that conditioned flavor of guilt may become a bit easier to handle, even if it continues to pop up.

Defensive reactions are also emotional messengers that can be difficult to interpret. Typically, we feel defensive when someone or something hits on an insecurity, or presses the bruises of past hurts or traumas. My client Mary really wanted a boyfriend. All her friends were in serious long-term relationships, and she felt envious. Over the phone, Mary's cousin asked her whether she had plans that weekend, and Mary's instant reaction was one of feeling judged. She snapped at her cousin, "Just because I'm single doesn't mean I never have plans!" Her cousin was flustered. She only wanted to see if Mary was available to have dinner. Yet because her cousin was married, and Mary was sensitive about her relationship status, she interpreted the innocent question as judgment laden. She treated her automatic feeling of insecurity as a messenger, bringing her the message that her cousin was judging her.

If she paused and considered the larger context of the situation, she would recognize that her cousin has never said or done anything to indicate she judges Mary for being single. It was Mary's own inner critic, plus her cultural conditioning, that made her feel embarrassed by her relationship status. Taking a pause and regulating herself in the face of emotional reactivity and defensiveness would have allowed her to more clearly discern what that emotion was about, and to choose with intention how she wished to respond in that specific situation, with that specific person.

We all feel defensive sometimes. In these situations, your emotion seems like it's cluing you into one thing, but really it's an indication of something else. As you practice listening to your emotions and getting clear on what they're telling you, it's important to take your time. If you're unsure what the emotion is communicating, or if it seems disproportionate or unrelated to the situation that elicited it, let it be. If there is truly a meaningful message underneath, it will present itself in due time.

There's one last thing to remember about emotions: sometimes they mean absolutely nothing! Your emotions can be influenced by life events, hormone levels, time of day, and any number of other biological, psychological, social, and environmental factors that you might not always be able to consciously pinpoint. Given their complexity, sometimes emotions will pop up that simply make no sense. You might just feel grumpy or irritable, even though the sun is shining, you're on vacation, you're well rested, fed, and have no clear reason to feel cranky. It happens! If you're not sure why a feeling is showing up, it's possible that there is no meaningful reason for it at all. If you leave it alone, you'll get through it much more easily than if you try to force a reason for it.

In her groundbreaking TED Talk *The Power of Vulnerability* (2010), Brené Brown reminded us that "we cannot selectively numb." It may be automatic for us to try to drown out unwanted emotions, but in doing so we also erode our ability to experience life's more enjoyable moments. Or, as the saying goes among ACT practitioners, we get so focused on feeling *good* that we forget how to *feel* good.

Being "good at feeling" means being able to notice what's there when it arises, without getting caught up in it. You notice what's happening in your body, and practice self-regulation if you're struggling to tolerate the feeling. Then, you can treat the feeling like a visiting guest. Greet it, and get curious about whether the guest is there to deliver a message. If the message isn't immediately clear, it's possible that it will present itself over time, or maybe there simply isn't a message accompanying this visitor. Regardless, you can rest assured that no matter how intense or overwhelming an emotional "guest" might be, it will always depart eventually.

If you're ever unsure how to handle an emotion or set of emotions, look to your values for guidance. Do your values tell you to ignore or suppress emotions until they leak out through passive-aggressive behavior? Do they tell you to silence yourself in order to please or accommodate others, even if you're secretly miserable as a result? Do they tell you to express your feelings in a way that hurts others, through hostility or aggression? You don't get to choose your emotions, but you do get to choose how you respond to them.

For those who value authenticity, self-silencing may not be the values-aligned way to respond to emotions because it would mean being fake. For those who value curiosity or self-awareness, numbing feelings would not be values aligned because it would prevent you from gaining the knowledge those feelings provide. For those who value kindness, lashing out at others would not be values aligned because you would be treating them cruelly.

For those who value connection, pretending everything is fine when your feelings are hurt would not be values aligned because being dishonest about your feelings would foster distance, not closeness, in the relationship. As you practice regulating yourself when feelings arise, you'll find that you can gain more from their messages and respond in ways that make you proud of yourself.

Your emotional world can provide wisdom about what you care about and what you need. When you tune in, you can use that wisdom meaningfully. Wellness and hustle cultures will tell you that some feelings are unacceptable and that you must silence yourself to preserve a certain image. Yet you can learn to stay rooted in your values and behave authentically even in the face of these pressures. *Intuition* is the ability to innately understand something without having to overanalyze. As you work on trusting your body, mind, and emotions to give you the information you need, you can begin to connect with the intuition that lives within you.

In the next section of this book, you'll learn to integrate sources of information from your mind, body, and context in order to live from a place of intuition. You'll prepare for potential challenges, whether from your own inner critic or from the outside world. Your intuition is like a compass, guiding you along your life's path. As you go, there will always be creatures that pop up to try to break your compass, or shake it up so that it's harder for you to read. Sometimes the creatures will come from your own mind, and other times they will come from the outside world. Our goal is to strengthen your inner compass, so that nothing can destroy it.

Your Unbreakable Inner Compass

PART 3

CHAPTER 10

Guided by Your Gut

Allie could hear her team members breaking down the latest episode of *The Bachelor* from down the hall. When she walked into the conference room, their animated chatter quieted. The truth was that Allie was also a *Bachelor* fan, but she never participated in these conversations. She believed that as their manager, she had to keep everyone focused, and if she let the conversation get too off topic her team wouldn't take her seriously. She felt pressure to present herself as confident and put-together. Meanwhile, her team members experienced her as cold and uptight. They got nervous when she put a meeting on their calendar, never knowing if she was going to point out a mistake with her matter-of-fact attitude. Allie's boss reinforced her leadership style, frequently reminding her that she needed to command respect from her team. She wasn't there to make friends, after all. Still, most days, Allie felt like she was acting—playing the part of a boss and tricking her staff into viewing her as an authority figure.

One morning, on her way into the building, a member of Allie's staff overheard her on the phone with a friend, cracking jokes about one of the *Bachelor* contestants. As they got on the elevator, the staffer said, "I didn't know you watched!" For a moment, Allie froze, worrying that she shouldn't be too friendly, but then she figured there was no harm in showing her personality. It was clear the young associate was eager to connect about their shared interest. They chatted about reality TV for a bit, then naturally segued into talking about some upcoming work projects. Outside of work, she was naturally bubbly and goofy, but after her promotion, she thought she had to keep that side of herself buttoned up. From that one interaction though, her corporate mask slipped off, and she could feel her whole body relax.

Allie realized that maybe the style of leadership that worked for her superiors wasn't authentic for her. She began to let her sense of humor come out with her team, and their responses surprised her. Instead of clamming up when she entered the room, they looked forward to her arrival. She took an interest in their lives, and in response, they felt like they could trust her and come to her for support.

Her anxiety about being respected began to ease. She discovered that if the conversation got off track, she could nudge everyone gently back to the task at hand, instead of coming down harshly in a way that never really vibed for her. By being herself and showing her humanity, she was still doing her job, but she was doing it authentically. Instead of playing the part of what she thought a boss was supposed to be, she was being the boss that only *she* could be. She was bringing her unique brand of enthusiasm, encouragement, and humor. Allie began leading from her intuition—trusting her knowledge and experience, considering the type of mentor she wanted to be, and listening to her body and emotions to guide her decision-making processes each day.

A few months into Allie's more authentic leadership style, she arrived one morning to find that Jose, the associate who was supposed to pitch to a big client, was nowhere to be found. She called his phone and he didn't answer. Something in her gut told her there was a problem. Instead of texting him a frantic *"You're late—where are you?!"* like she would have in the past, she texted, *"Is everything okay?"* and then asked another associate to prepare to take over the pitch.

When she finally heard from Jose an hour later, she answered him with genuine relief. Sure enough, her gut had been correct. Jose's mom had a heart attack that morning and he had rushed with her to the emergency room. The old Allie would have been so fixated on being the boss that she would have jumped to conclusions. When she saw Jose was missing on a big day, she would've called him to angrily demand an explanation. Instead, from this new authentic place, she was able to listen to her gut. It was unlike Jose to run late without communicating. She instinctively integrated knowledge about the situation and context, her inner thoughts and feelings, and her values of kindness and respect, to decide how to behave in the heat of the moment.

When you're operating from a place of authenticity, you have this same ability to instinctively use information from your mind, body, and the situational context to decide how to behave. You have the capacity to think critically—not only about the messages swirling in the culture around you, but also about the messages being sent from your own mind and body. You also have an awareness of your true values, and an understanding of how those values can guide you in your daily life. The rest of this book will help you integrate all these sources of information so that they come together in a cohesive and helpful way. When you're connected to your mind, body, emotions, and personal values, you hone that deeper gut sense—your intuition. Living from your intuition is like having an inner compass that guides you, sometimes in the span of a single instant, to *just know* where to go or what to do.

The outside world tries to sell you a replacement for intuition. The ideals of wellness and hustle cultures seem like they provide a clear evaluation of whether you're doing it "right." Eat this, not that. Do this amount of exercise. Take these supplements, use this bullet journal. Doing these things can feel like you're doing something right. Measurements like grades, performance reports, and billable hours can provide a false sense of comfort. If you're ever unsure what to do, you can always turn to the outside world. Someone out there will be happy to tell you what to do, insisting there is a correct choice. These cultural forces are so powerful (and that hit of dopamine you get from receiving approval is so alluring) that you might come to believe that other people know better than you about what you need.

Conversely, if you're not guided by those rules and mandates, everyday decision making can feel daunting. We face countless decisions every day that don't have an objective right or wrong answer. How do you know whether to break up with the person you're dating, or move to a new city, or stay at your current job? These aren't decisions anyone else can make for you. If you surveyed a hundred people you would likely get a hundred different answers—and all might be right for someone. Yet the only person who knows the right answer for you, in your unique life and situation, is *you*. Now that you have a clearer sense of your own values, it might be time to focus less on whether you're doing things right, and more on whether you're doing things in a way that's right for you. Shifting from the pursuit of "right" to the pursuit of "authentic" comes from listening to your gut.

Of course, even if you're in the habit of making decisions based on intuition, you still won't have complete freedom over the direction of your life. While everyone deserves autonomy, many decisions are taken away from people due to systemic inequalities and circumstances beyond individual control. Opportunities aren't available to everyone equally. Still, even in situations where your choices are extremely limited, you have control over your own behavior. You don't choose what happens to you, but you do choose how to respond. Every day, you face decisions of varying significance, whether you're figuring out when to seek medical care for a symptom, when to say "I love you" for the first time, how to recover after making a mistake, or how to handle hurt feelings. You may not consciously or logically know what to do in these moments, but deep down in your gut, the answer awaits. You can't think your way to it or force it out; you have to open up, give it time, and trust it to arrive.

For years, my incredibly patient therapist tried to connect me to my gut. I'd sit on her couch agonizing over decisions big and small, weighing pros and cons of every possible move I could make. I'd fixate on how others would react to my choices, or what I felt like I "should" do, and wallow in despair. I insisted that I didn't know what to do. "Yes, you do. Drop down into your body," she'd say. I'd close my eyes and try to check my gut, but it felt impossible. Then I'd get frustrated and repeat the cycle: fixate, agonize, beat myself up for not figuring it out. "Give it time," she'd say. "You'll know the answer when there is one." Finally, I had an experience where it all clicked: when my intuition told me I had found the person who would become my partner.

I met Jeremy when I was nineteen and he was twenty-two, working as camp counselors one summer. When summer ended and we went our separate ways, he wanted to pursue a long-distance relationship, but I put him in the friend zone. He was *so nice*, so consistent, and the unhealed part of me didn't know how to handle his stability. Over the course of the next decade, I had a string of relationships with people who charmed and excited me but were ultimately emotionally unavailable. Eventually, with the help of that same gut-guiding therapist, I learned that I needed a partner who was secure and consistent. I set off to meet someone who wouldn't get skittish when I cried or act annoyed when I expressed myself, who made me feel genuinely respected. It didn't occur to me that I had already met someone who did exactly that.

One night in my late twenties, I was at home listening to music and stretching on my yoga mat. A song came on that reminded me of that summer at camp, and I began to reminisce. Jeremy's face popped into my head for the first time in a few years. I thought, *I wonder how he's doing these days*, and sent him a text.

The next day we got on the phone and before we knew it, we'd been talking for hours. We decided he would fly to town to visit me the following weekend. I was nervous, but as soon as I saw him, I felt a sense of calm. We spent the weekend catching up. I was surprised to discover that the self-consciousness I usually felt while dating was absent. Something in my gut said, *This is right*. There was no intense burst of fireworks, but there also wasn't a "will we, won't we" tug-of-war in my brain. There was a calm little gut feeling telling me to go forward, and that quiet confidence grew stronger each time we saw each other.

You may be able to recall moments similar to this one, where you just instinctively knew something was right or something needed to be done. It could be that you knew when it was time to end a relationship, put an offer on a house, or look for a new job. You might be able to tell when your child is getting sick, or when it's time to say good-bye to a pet. On a smaller scale, it comes in the form of knowing what to have for dinner that will leave you feeling exactly as satisfied as you want, or when a friend could use a little pick-me-up. Intuition doesn't come from the outside world, but it also doesn't operate in a vacuum. You might learn things from the people around you or gather context clues, and still that gut instinct comes from within. Sometimes it can even feel like a spiritual signal, a deep sense of knowing.

Sadly, our gut instinct is not always cultivated. When you're repeatedly discouraged from listening to your gut, it's easy to get caught up in over-analysis and decision paralysis. Or you can become impulsive, only chasing things that feel good without diving deeper to find out if something else is more authentic for you. While intuition itself is more of an instinct than something you can think your way through, for someone who has been disconnected from their gut for a long time it can help to have some steps to follow while you work on reconnecting. You might think of the following process as a sort of blueprint for honing intuition:

1. Tune in to your mental, physical, and emotional signals. What cues are happening in your body, what emotions are you experiencing, and what are the thoughts going through your mind?

2. Consider what those signals are telling you. Use the curious, observational attitude you've honed throughout this book, and try to notice those signals without jumping to conclusions.

3. Consider your context and any relevant information from the outside world. Does your immediate reaction make sense based on where you are, who you're with, what you're doing, or your awareness of previous similar situations? Are there potential consequences to your decision that you need to consider?

4. Consider any prominent physical, psychological, social, or spiritual needs.

5. Keep your values at the forefront. Use them to guide you toward a response to those prominent needs.

This might seem like heady work; if every time you had a decision to make, you had to break it into a five-step process, it would be hard to get much done. No worries—with practice and regular attunement, the process begins to feel more instinctive.

Like driving a car, you might start off fixating on each step of the process until you're practiced enough that it becomes automatic. Most new drivers have some degree of anxiety over the minutiae of operating a vehicle, so their brains might go something like this: *Did I adjust the rear-view mirror? Okay, let me shift to reverse now. Which way for the right-turn signal and which for the left again? Whoops, I'm going over the speed limit, better slow down.* Once you've gotten behind the wheel enough times, your confidence grows and that mental chatter disappears. Then one day, you're just driving. You're still attuned to those little details, but without as much conscious effort. Once you've been tuning in to your inner world for a while, the "knowing what to do" part of decision making becomes more instinctual.

Attending to Your Needs

One aspect of honing intuition is knowing when you have a strong need. Needs get a bad reputation among the people-pleasing crowd, since we're often taught to associate needs with being self-indulgent or entitled. But by virtue of being alive, all humans have needs, and many of those needs are actually more altruistic than self-serving. Psychologist Alfred Adler popularized the idea that humans have a need to contribute to their community or society, and we are most psychologically healthy when we feel a sense of belongingness (Adler 2010).

While there are some needs we all share, like basic survival needs for food, water, air, and shelter, there are other psychological, social, emotional, and spiritual needs that differ from person to person. You may have an especially strong need for intellectual stimulation, while someone else may have a particularly strong need for creative expression.

You might also learn that some needs pop up pretty regularly, while others are at the forefront only every once in a while. A need that isn't usually prominent can emerge at a given time. Maybe when you're going through a painful life event like losing a loved one, you have a higher need for physical touch. Maybe if you've just lost your job, you have a stronger need for reassurance than usual. At certain points in time, you might feel a strong need to contribute or offer support to others, while at other times you might need to conserve your energy. Like most things in life, it depends on the context. When you're familiar with your needs and know how to attend to them, you're in a strong position to recognize when something feels off and to shift direction.

At http://www.newharbinger.com/54063, you'll find an inventory of needs across various domains, created by the Center for Nonviolent Communication. This inventory can help you gain insight into which needs you might be facing right now, and which ones tend to be most significant for you. As you read the inventory, write down or circle the needs you currently have that are being met, or that you know you can easily meet. Next, write down or highlight the needs you currently have that aren't regularly met. Finally, what are some things that would help you attend to those unmet needs?

Tuning In to Your Intuition

When you tune in, your intuition guides you in the direction that is right for you. Sometimes it acts like a GPS, efficiently bringing you to a precise location. That happens when you immediately know *exactly* what you need or what to do. Your friend falls and appears to be having a seizure, and you instantly grab your phone to dial 911. In other situations, it's more like an old-school compass, pointing you in enough of a general direction to know you're not lost, but the precision of where you land unfolds more slowly, over the course of time. That happens when you know what you want to study in school, but aren't quite sure what position you'll want to take in that field of study once you graduate. Sometimes, intuition feels more like an educated guess than a confident yes, so don't panic if you have a general gut sense of something but you aren't quite certain about the specifics.

Trusting your intuition is not about ignoring logic or acting impulsively. It's actually quite the opposite—guiding you to take committed action based on the things that matter to you, taking into consideration the information from your mind and body in the process. As you practice going inside for answers, your gut instincts may become louder and more automatic. Sometimes the answers won't appear when you want them to. You'll feel completely lost and unsure whether you're moving in the right direction, only to discover as you go along that you're either on the right track, or you'd be well served to change course. You can hone your intuition by regularly reminding yourself of your values, watching your thoughts with curiosity, responding to whatever signals your body is sending you, and noticing any messages underneath your emotions. When you regularly tune in to these different channels of communication that live inside you, your gut instinct gets easier to spot and follow.

One way to strengthen the connection is through the ACT process of *committed action*. In any given situation, you have choices about how to behave. Commitment is about choosing to act in alignment with your values, over and over again. It involves not only a strong sense of dedication to your values but also flexibility to modify what you do based on what the situation calls for and what is available to you.

My client Ariel has a core value of compassion. When complaining about a pushy coworker who was irritating her, she caught herself and said, "I'm frustrated, but I can empathize with her. I guess I'd be pushy too if I had a child with cancer. She probably has to advocate for him constantly." That quick reconnection to her value of compassion helped her change her behavior in the moment. She had been complaining and criticizing someone, which felt off to her gut. She realized she was not behaving compassionately. With awareness, she recommitted to behaving with compassion. After many more moments like this where she noticed herself behaving judgmentally and shifted to compassion, Ariel eventually noticed that her first thought when someone annoyed her was *Wow, I bet they have a lot going on*, instead of immediately criticizing them. Continuously committing to compassion allowed her to more automatically respond to situations in ways that were authentic to her. She didn't invalidate her feeling of annoyance when it arose, but she chose to respond to that feeling by refocusing on behaving in a values-aligned way.

Acting Authentically

You can use your journal or download this activity at http://www.newhar binger.com/54063. Write down one of your top values that you identified in chapter 5.

Now, write about a situation where you *didn't* act in alignment with that value.

What could you have done differently to behave in a way that was more congruent with your value?

Consider a situation in which you *did* act according to that value. What did you say, do, or focus on?

What commitment can you make today regarding how you want to behave in similar situations?

Given how prescriptive and commanding the dominant culture can be, it's hard to peel away the layers of conditioning to connect with your gut instinct. Sometimes you'll have to go through a discernment process much like you do when determining whether an emotion is a valuable messenger or a conditioned reaction. This is especially necessary when your gut tells you something that goes against what you've been taught to do. Maybe you learned to always be polite and never make other people (especially men) uncomfortable. If that's the case, your gut might tell you to say no to a drink with a pushy stranger who violates your personal space, but that conditioned part of you might feel guilty for doing so. Maybe you learned to be helpful and accommodating, so saying no when your friend asks for a ride to the airport on a day where you have too much else going on might evoke guilt, despite knowing in your gut that you simply cannot do this favor. It can help to remember that trusting your gut isn't about just doing whatever you want. Your intuition comes from a protective, instinctive place, and sometimes protecting yourself or honoring your values involves doing something that upsets another person.

As you continue committing to your values and acting in alignment with them, it will get easier to trust your gut even when it goes against socially prescribed expectations. The more you show up authentically, the more opportunities you'll have to discover whether you like being this way. Your gut will start to develop a track record of steering you in the direction that's right for you.

However, you'll still encounter situations every day where you must choose between acting authentically and honoring your values, or acting in a way that aligns with the values set forth by wellness or hustle cultures. These situations will shine a light on where you might need to create or uphold boundaries in your life. There might be people who don't respect your needs or decisions. You might discover that some of your relationships have been built on a false sense of shared values, where the other person values things that you were taught to care about but now realize you don't truly care about.

In the next chapter, we'll explore assertive communication and boundary setting, so that you can go about your life confident in your ability to carve your own path. Boundaries are there to protect, not shut out. When you set them in authentic ways, you'll discover that effective boundaries actually enhance your relationships.

CHAPTER 11

Building Better Boundaries

Tanya was known at work as the ultimate team player. If someone needed their shift covered, they knew to ask her before anyone else. Even though she was constantly saying yes, she still felt like she was always letting someone down. If she agreed to cover an extra shift, her boyfriend got upset that she was missing their date night. If she agreed to drive a friend to the airport on a Sunday night, her mother would be disappointed that she couldn't come over for Sunday dinner. Logically, she knew that if she didn't agree to these favors, people would figure out another solution, but she still felt guilty if she couldn't make every one happy.

Tanya's family, friends, and coworkers were so used to hearing yes that they didn't realize they were taking advantage of her. They sometimes acted entitled to her time or energy. She was often treated like her needs were less important than everyone else's. She vacillated between guilt for not being able to make everyone happy, and resentment that nobody ever asked what *she* wanted. Most of the time, she genuinely enjoyed helping people, but she didn't always have the energy or resources for it. Tanya thought she needed an extra six hours in her day to better accommodate everyone, but what she really needed were some clearly stated boundaries.

Like Tanya, some of us are conditioned to believe that we should always agree with others and go along with their wishes. We believe it's our job to make others happy, even if it comes at our own expense. This mentality lends itself to a passive communication style. Other people learn the opposite—that they must compete constantly, and that winning or being in the dominant position is the most important thing. This belief system lends itself to an aggressive communication style. Neither of these approaches tends to be satisfying, because they involve either denying your own needs or denying other people's. Some people try to find a workaround. They want to honor their needs and preferences, but don't know how, so they try to do so in a more roundabout and indirect way, using a passive-aggressive communication style. Passive-aggressiveness is hard to call out because it's not obvious aggression, but it comes across as defensive or inauthentic.

There's a fourth option. This option involves being calm, respectful, and direct—in other words, assertive. Assertive communication demonstrates respect for both your own needs and the other person's needs. If you're being assertive, you're expressing your needs clearly, without implying that the other person's needs don't matter. As the cliche goes, a relationship is a two-way street. In a healthy dynamic, both people recognize values differences and communicate assertively to find compromises that respect both parties and preserve the relationship.

Boundary setting is a cornerstone of assertive communication. A boundary is a limit around what you will or will not do, and what you are and aren't comfortable with. In a culture that glorifies productivity and doing it all, boundary setting is not always a well-practiced skill. Yet boundaries are some of the most important tools for creating fulfilling relationships with our friends, family, and others, and with the surrounding culture. By setting effective boundaries, you can protect yourself from succumbing to pressures from toxic systems. You can ensure you won't go back to the striving that burned you out in the first place.

A lot of people are afraid that setting boundaries will push away those they love. You may worry that people won't like your boundaries, and the idea of someone being mad at you seems unbearable. Here's the thing: the people who are most upset about your boundaries, or who give you a hard time for setting them, are likely to be the people who benefit from you being a doormat. In a supportive, mutually respectful relationship, there is room for both parties to have needs and preferences. In these relationships, effective boundaries do not shut out the other person; rather, they provide guardrails that ensure safety and build trust. Boundaries allow the relationship to be contained in a way that enhances both people's lives.

When one person changes and the other person doesn't, a relationship may go through growing pains. This is where boundary setting is crucial, whether to inform the other person of your new set of priorities, or to take some space if it's unhealthy for you to be close to that person in any capacity. Maybe some of the people you were close with while entrenched in wellness culture are still focused on ideals you no longer share. If your friendship was built upon sharing diet tips, trying the latest cleanse together, or keeping each other accountable for workouts, you may discover that without those topics, you don't have much else in common. Or maybe you have friends who reinforce hustle culture, pushing you to ignore your limits, bragging about how many tasks they accomplished today or making you feel judged for taking a vacation.

Boundaries allow you to maintain alignment with your personal values. Perhaps you committed to attending a friend's big gallery opening, which aligns with your values of friendship and supportiveness. Then your boss asks you to stay late to finish a task that you could easily do tomorrow. If you don't set a boundary, you'll have to miss the opening, and will behave in a way that pleases your boss, but goes against the type of friend you want to be. Context is key. Sometimes, boundaries are tricky because your values conflict with one another. Maybe in the same scenario, you struggle to choose a course of action because you hold values of friendship, supportiveness, and cooperation. In these situations where your values conflict, you might have to decide which one is most important in that specific moment, and set a boundary accordingly.

How to Set a Boundary

A few years ago, I unexpectedly went viral on TikTok with a video about setting boundaries in the face of judgmental or intrusive comments. While I am famously late to most trends, I was ahead of the curve on this one. Nowadays, you can find hundreds of thousands of videos on #boundaries, but like a lot of what you encounter online, not every "how to set a boundary" post contains accurate information. A key element of boundaries that gets lost in the sea of hot takes and pithy one-liners is that they are meant to protect relationships. Their purpose is not to have the last word or to put someone in their place. Their purpose is to make your needs known so that the other person is aware of how you wish to be treated in order for the relationship to thrive. These tips can help you accomplish this:

Use "I" statements. When you lead with the word "you," it can land as an attack even if the request itself seems reasonable. People don't like being told what to do. By making the same request with an emphasis on what "I need" and "I feel," you have a better chance of being heard accurately. Plus, you can't tell other people what's true about them, but you can tell them what's true about you. "You're being mean" is something they can deny ("What are you talking about? No, I'm not!") but "I feel disrespected" is not something they can argue with, because they can't tell you whether you feel that way or not.

Focus on specific behavior. Boundaries are most effective when they can be clearly measured and observed. Something like "Please don't be rude to me" can come across as confusing because it's vague. What you consider rude may not match someone else's definition. Instead, pointing to specific actions, such as "Please don't interrupt me when I'm speaking," or "Please speak to me in a lower volume" will paint a much clearer picture of what you're seeking and leave less room for misinterpretation. One effective boundary format is to combine an "I" statement with a request for behavior change as follows: "When you (*name specific behavior*), I feel (*name specific feeling*). Please (*name specific behavior you would like them to do instead*)."

Identify what you'll do if the boundary is not respected. When you ask someone to respect a boundary, they may or may not honor your request. If they do, that's wonderful. If they don't, you can reiterate it by repeating the original request along with information about what you plan to do if it is violated again. For instance, if your mom ignores your clearly stated boundary of "Please don't comment on my weight," you might need to add a consequence: "Please don't comment on my weight. If you comment on my weight again, I'm going to leave the room/end the conversation/stop coming over for dinner." Just make sure that any consequence you're asserting is something you actually plan to do. Otherwise, you risk the other person learning that your words are empty; they can continue to get away with disrespectful behavior without consequence.

Give the person an opportunity to change their behavior. A boundary can't be respected if the other person doesn't know about it. Your boundary might seem obvious to you, but the other person may be learning for the first time that their behavior bothers you. Most people—especially those who care about you—aren't trying to hurt you on purpose. Relationships tend to be more satisfying when both parties assume positive intent from the other person. It's your choice whether or not you want to give someone the chance to correct the course. You certainly aren't obligated to keep someone in your life when they've hurt you. However, you may end up pretty isolated, if you make a habit of cutting people off before they've had a chance to try showing up differently.

Be open to feedback. Just as you're entitled to set boundaries, so are other people. If you can take others' feedback nondefensively, and respect their boundaries, you'll demonstrate that you see relationships as two-way streets. Relationships involve negotiating differences in each party's needs. You don't have to understand or agree with a boundary in order to respect it. If your brother says he can visit for only an hour, and you wish he could stay longer, you can feel disappointed (and even express that disappointment) *without* disrespecting his boundary. He has a right to set limits on his behavior, just as you have that same right. You have to decide whether you'd rather have him come for only an hour or not at all. Sometimes you may accept a boundary even if you dislike it, because it allows you to have a relationship with the other person.

There will inevitably be people in your life who don't respect your boundaries. Although most of us have some degree of choice in the company we keep, there will always be "necessary evils," people you wouldn't choose but are stuck with. Sometimes it's an intrusive coworker you have to work beside each day, a nosy neighbor, or a relative you can't completely avoid at the holidays. While *technically* you could find a new job, move to a new neighborhood, or skip family events, the lengths you'd have to take to com- pletely avoid these individuals may be too detrimental to your well-being. Thus, when you're required to engage with people who reinforce harmful ideas or treat you in ways that don't align with your values, remember that you have control over your own side. You can do everything in your power to minimize contact with those people and choose how much attention and importance to attach to their actions and opinions. You can choose whether to take them seriously, or with a grain of salt.

People don't stay exactly the same over time. Our priorities and preferences shift as we move through life, so boundaries will need to be adjusted accordingly. At some points in time, it may be harmful to you to be close with a certain person, while at other times, you find that you're enjoying your interactions with that same person. There will be seasons in your life where you gravitate toward certain friends, and other times where those relationships naturally fade out. However, there are occasionally situations where the safest boundary you can set is to completely end contact.

If someone has harmed or abused you, you're not obligated to keep them in your life. When someone has a history of behaving in a way that is abusive or violent, it might put you in further danger to attempt to set boundaries through assertive communication. If you're worried about your safety in any relationship, please do not attempt to use the strategies from this chapter to engage with them. Instead, seek support from a trained mental health professional or law enforcement authority to ensure you can safely end the relationship.

Note: *If you or someone you know is the victim of domestic violence or abuse, you can call the National Domestic Violence Hotline at 800-799-7233 or visit thehotline.org for help.*

In other situations, someone might not be physically violent, but may have repeatedly and blatantly violated your boundaries. Here, you might also choose to go no-contact. This can be a complicated decision to make, especially if the individual in question is a family member. Despite what you may have been taught, you're not obligated to keep someone in your life if they treat you in ways that are disrespectful, especially if you have attempted to set boundaries with them or assert yourself and they have continued to disregard your well-being. If you're struggling with the decision, it can be helpful to consult with a trusted confidante or trained mental health professional. Only you can decide whether ending a relationship is the best choice for you, and whether it aligns with your values to do so.

Boundary Setting 101

You can do this activity in your journal or download it at http://www
.newharbinger.com/54063. Describe a situation where you would like to set
better boundaries. Talk about the person or people involved, the way they
usually behave, the way you usually behave, and what exactly you want to
be different.

Now, using the tips you've learned in this chapter, craft a boundary
that applies to this situation you identified:

How do you feel when you imagine setting the boundary you outlined
here? Name any fears, hopes, and potential obstacles.

What could help you overcome these obstacles?

If you're not ready to set this boundary, commit to rehearsing it with a
trusted friend or therapist. Practicing can help you "try on" what it might
be like to communicate in a direct, self-respecting manner, until you feel
ready to give it a shot.

If you were conditioned as a child to self-silence to avoid upsetting
others, it can be hard to recognize that you might play a role in upholding
passive or passive-aggressive dynamics in your adult life. This doesn't mean
it's your fault if people are disrespectful to you. You should always be treated
with respect, and you shouldn't have to ask for it. Yet sometimes, when
you're accustomed to passivity and fear, you might not treat *yourself* with
the respect you deserve. This can also make it hard to recognize when the
other person is giving you signs that they *do* respect you. You might inadvertently project assumptions onto them or misinterpret their behavior as
aggressive. With greater awareness, you can begin to heal from past mis-
treatment so you don't repeat hurtful patterns. You can begin to assert
yourself unapologetically, and let yourself receive care and respect from
others when they offer it.

Tiana and her partner Rae were stuck in a dynamic that highlights
how self-silencing can interfere with a loving relationship. Tiana grew up
with a father who frequently screamed at her, and she developed a passive
communication style. Although Rae was typically assertive and direct,
Tiana often braced herself and expected explosive outbursts. When Tiana

needed their home office for a work call and Rae was already in there reading, Tiana would qualify her requests with excessive apologies. She'd timidly knock on the door, eyes downcast, and mumble, "Um, if it's okay with you, I'm so sorry but I have a work call that I need to take in here. I'm so sorry, I know it's so annoying to have to move." Rae would get upset because she felt like Tiana perceived her as a ticking time bomb, despite her track record of generally behaving in ways that were calm and respectful.

One day, as Tiana slunk into the room to ask a favor, Rae voiced her frustration. She said, "Tiana, why do you assume I'm going to explode if you ask me to move rooms? If you tell me what you want, I promise I'll listen. But when you tiptoe around me, it makes me feel like you think I'm some monster. Even if I'm sometimes annoyed about moving rooms, I'm not going to yell at you."

Tiana realized that she was assuming that Rae—and everyone else— would be intolerant if she ever expressed needs, because that's how her father reacted. But not everyone was her father. In fact, making herself small and unobtrusive might have protected her as a child, but as an adult, her passivity was actually interfering with her desire for reciprocal, mutually respectful relationships. Rae made it clear that even if she *did* get annoyed sometimes, that didn't mean Tiana wasn't allowed to assert herself, and it didn't change how Rae felt about her. Their relationship was strong enough to handle temporary feelings of frustration.

Tiana realized she wanted to teach people to treat her as an equal. Instead of letting the other person decide whether they felt she deserved respect, she began to enter interactions under the assumption that she (and they) automatically deserved respect. Starting with Rae, whom she knew she could trust, she practiced showing self-respect. She began making requests with direct eye contact, relaxed body language, and assertive state- ments. While she still encountered people who were rude or belittling, Tiana knew she deserved better. Instead of making it her job to prevent the other person from getting explosive, she saw others as responsible for their own behavior. Becoming more assertive helped Tiana take back her power and show up in the world in a way that demonstrated the belief that she— and everyone else—deserved respect. This also helped her gravitate toward friendships with people who treated her with respect, instead of finding herself in familiar but painful dynamics with so-called friends who replicated the aggressive behavior she grew up around.

Setting Boundaries with What You Consume

Even if you surround yourself with people who share your values and don't expect unquestioning obedience, you still can't escape systemic messaging. Sometimes, just turning on the TV or seeing a billboard on the road, you'll be reminded of societal pressures. Unless you go live in a bubble and never leave the house or interact with another human being ever again, you can't completely avoid toxic messaging. A great way to handle these messages is to enhance your media literacy, which involves "interrogat[ing] the choices and messages made by companies and individuals to determine what is true and what is false; what preys on your insecurities and attempts to manipulate your reality versus what serves you" (Kite and Kite 2024).

Regularly asking yourself how you feel when you consume various types of content can help you identify where you might need boundaries. A boundary might involve limiting or completely stopping exposure to that particular source of media when possible, or minimizing the amount of attention you focus on that content, if it's not possible to avoid.

Here are some ways you could set boundaries with media:

- Limiting use of electronics (or limiting time spent on social media) to certain hours of the day, or setting a media "curfew" where you unplug during certain times of the day

- Having one day per week or one hour per day where you do a complete media blackout, not using devices or going online unless absolutely necessary

- Unfollowing or muting social media accounts that have a negative effect on your well-being or influence you to behave in ways that don't match your values

- Unfollowing or muting social media accounts that lead to body or appearance-based comparisons, or comparisons about your productivity or accomplishments

- If it's important to you to be informed about current events, being intentional to do so in a contained, specific way (for example, reading a synopsis each morning from a trusted news outlet, then turning it off for the rest of the day...or going old school and reading the newspaper!)

By being intentional about the way you engage with external messaging, you can set boundaries that protect your well-being and allow you to stay connected with the priorities and ideals you find most meaningful. Decreasing your engagement with messaging that takes you away from your values or causes you to ruminate on unhelpful ideas can make a huge difference for your well-being. You can also intentionally expose yourself to messaging that is values aligned for you, in an effort to influence yourself in a positive way. You can't control what's out there, but you can choose what you consume, and what you create, share, and amplify on social media.

Most media messaging is meant to influence you in some way, whether to buy a product or simply to continue spending time on that platform long enough to be served more ads. Dr. Cal Newport (2019) describes this system as "the attention economy." Your attention is the precious resource companies are vying for. The goal of most apps and social media platforms is to keep the user on them as long as possible, and they accomplish this with increasingly sophisticated algorithms. The longer these companies can keep you engaged or scrolling, the more opportunities they have to influence what you care about. If you're wise to it, you can refuse to let your focus get hijacked, and instead be intentional about where you put your energy.

As you practice setting boundaries with the people and systems around you, you might discover that assertiveness gets easier. You may never be someone who enjoys standing up for yourself, but you'll get better at tolerating the discomfort that arises in those scenarios. Remember that you're just as worthy of respect as everyone else. Asserting yourself and setting boundaries does not guarantee that you'll always be treated with respect, or that you'll get the desired results. Regardless, asserting yourself is an exercise in self-respect and empowerment. Even if you don't always get the response you hope for, being assertive ensures you'll be happy with how you behaved. You can walk away from the situation knowing you stood up for yourself in a way that was firm but respectful. You weren't a doormat, but you also weren't domineering.

Regular boundary setting can make you more resilient in the face of cultural pressures. Those messages will continue to swirl, but you'll be less susceptible to their influence. You're more than a pawn in the dominant culture's agenda. You're more than an object to be looked at or consumed. You're not on this planet just to serve others, even if helpfulness or compassion are core values of yours. You're also allowed to evolve and change from one day to the next and one moment to the next. Those changes can happen in physical form as your body shifts and morphs throughout life, and those changes can happen in your preferences, needs, emotional states, priorities, and personality traits. Although it is often meaningful to develop a cohesive identity, it is also important not to get too attached to any one aspect of yourself.

In the next chapter, you'll learn to make shifts in self-perception so that you can build more flexibility. Instead of clinging tightly to any one idea about yourself or your body, you can make space for the fluidity of your experience on this planet.

CHAPTER 12

Bigger Than Your Body

Sixteen-year-old Elena sprawled on her bed, phone in hand, and clicked open her Facetune app. She uploaded a photo of herself in a bikini from a recent family vacation and got to work. After using tools to scoop and reshape her stomach, perk up her butt, slim her thighs, bronze her skin, lift her cheekbones, and make her hair smoother and shinier, she was satisfied. She sent the result to her best friend, who texted back, "OMG, you look like a Kardashian!" She then posted the picture on Instagram where, within minutes, her feed lit up with fire emojis. All of her friends edited their photos beyond recognition. Elena wondered if she could ever sculpt her body like this in real life if she found the right workout, diet, or surgery. For now, the photos were aspirational, an escapist fantasy for when she was feeling bad about herself.

Down the hall, Elena's mother scowled at herself in the bathroom mirror, pinching at the rolls on her stomach and pushing her breasts up higher on her chest, closer to where they were fifteen years ago. She'd hated her body when her stomach was tighter and her breasts sat higher, too. If only she'd realized back then that she was beautiful, she lamented. After three kids and now, in early menopause, her body looked nothing like it had in her twenties. Her skin dimpled and sagged where it used to be smooth. Her eyes had new crinkles around them, and her hair was becoming more gray than brown each day. Sometimes she found it easier to avoid mirrors completely. Other days, like today, she stood close to her reflection and picked herself apart. She hated herself for it. She felt simultaneously superficial for caring, and miserable because she just wanted to feel attractive.

The coauthors of *Intuitive Eating* remind us, "Just as a person with a shoe size of eight would not expect to realistically squeeze into a size six, it is equally futile (and uncomfortable) to have the same expectation about body size" (Tribole and Resch 2020). To liken it to another life form, nobody expects an oak tree to resemble a palm tree, or for a tree to look the same as it did in its youth. Whether it's an oak, elm, or apple tree, the tree begins as a seed, growing into a sapling. Even once mature, a tree continues to change. New buds in the spring become flowers. Leaves change color, dry up, and fall to the ground each autumn. Just like nobody blames an oak for not being a palm, nobody blames a tree for changing with each passing moment either. In fact, people often marvel at the unique beauty that arrives with a new season.

All living creatures look different from one another, *and* different from previous versions of themselves as time goes on. For some reason, only humans (especially humans socialized as female) are expected to conform to a specific aesthetic, and then freeze time at a certain point, attaining and then maintaining a rigid beauty standard from birth until death. We rage against the natural fluidity and diversity of being alive, attempting to force ourselves into submissive conformity. There is an acceptable way to look, and we're not supposed to deviate from it, regardless of any natural diversity among us, and regardless of our movement through various seasons of life.

Entire industries are built on these rigid ideals. We're sold products to reverse the effects of aging, childbirth, menopause, and any other natural life experience. Wrinkles, stretch marks, weight gain, and graying hair are seen as problems to solve, indications that we've let ourselves go. Even if you fit the mold at one point, you'll have to keep up with changing trends. One day the goal is to be as thin as possible, while the next day it's big boobs, a big butt, and muscular legs. No matter how hard we try, we never feel attractive for long. Beauty standards are created based on whatever is hardest to attain, so it's only a matter of time before they change. It's understandable to want to achieve beauty standards. Society is not kind to those who don't match up. Ageism, colorism, fatphobia, and transphobia are prime examples of socially constructed inequities that punish those who don't fit the dominant system's version of acceptable appearance.

Most body-based anxieties are rooted in fatphobia and result from weight stigma. My client Theresa was painfully, intimately familiar with this reality. Theresa had lived in a larger body for her entire life. She had the same build as all the women in her family. For as long as she could remember, she'd been told her body was wrong. In elementary school, her PE teacher made her run extra laps. Theresa learned to use exercise to punish her body for its size and shape. She became obsessed with fitness, and in college became certified to teach yoga and spin classes. Still, when she'd enter the gym, there were people who didn't believe she was the instructor; they assumed she was a new student.

Every doctor she ever saw told her she needed to lose weight, without bothering to ask about her eating or exercise habits, and usually ignoring whatever complaint had brought her to seek their care in the first place. Everything was blamed on her weight, and she was made to feel that any hardship she faced was her own fault. If she was bruised from squeezing into chairs that were too small for her body, it was her body's fault for not being smaller. If she was suffering from knee pain, it was automatically blamed on her weight, despite evidence that the pain could be nerve damage from a recent car accident. At the grocery store, strangers commented on what was in her cart. Given how she was treated, it was no surprise that Theresa developed a raging eating disorder that went undiagnosed for over two decades.

When Theresa discovered a size-inclusive yoga studio in her early thirties, she felt like she'd entered a different universe. In this space, bodies of all shapes, sizes, ages, and abilities were honored. There were no mirrors, and no comments about shredding or toning. The instructors offered various props and modifications to help make shapes and movements more accessible to each student. The studio became Theresa's refuge. Soon she'd built a community around her of people in diverse bodies, people who celebrated their bodies instead of punishing them for not complying with harsh societal ideals. Her new friends introduced her to size-inclusive fitness brands and clothing, and the fat-positive movement. She was able to find new health care providers who identified as weight neutral and actually listened to her concerns instead of prescribing weight loss. She began therapy to heal her eating disorder.

Many years later, Theresa became an advocate for size inclusivity in fitness. She started speaking at local gyms and yoga studios, advising them on how to make changes to their programming and facilities so that people in larger bodies would feel more welcome and comfortable. The world around Theresa remained entrenched in weight bias, and she continued to face barriers in her everyday life. Yet she no longer believed her body was a problem. She now knew the problems to solve were societal. She came to understand deep down that her body deserved—and had *always* been worthy of—unconditional respect. This is one of the core principles of the intuitive eating model and the heart of the ™ (HAES) philosophy (Bacon 2008; Burgard 2009; Tribole and Resch 2020; Tylka et al. 2014). You deserve to accept your body and honor it by nourishing it, clothing it, and treating it with kindness. This is *always* true. Your body deserves dignity exactly as it is today, even if it isn't how you think it should be, and even if it's different from how it used to be.

Wellness culture and its partner in crime, diet culture, love to attach desirable attributes to an aesthetic. Without realizing it, you unconsciously absorb and buy into appearance-based biases, even if logically you don't really think someone is smarter, more competent, or superior for how they look. In psychology, we call this the halo effect. If we don't know much about someone, we make assumptions based on whatever information we have. When the information is positive, we assume other positive things about that person. When someone fits a cultural beauty standard, we register this as positive and assume that the attractive person possesses other positive qualities and characteristics (Talamas, Mavor, and Perrett 2016).

When people automatically assume you possess positive traits, it's a lot easier to move through the world. Given the privilege that comes with fitting society's beauty standards, it's understandable to want to fit those standards. But just as Theresa discovered, although it's more difficult, it is entirely possible to find fulfillment in your everyday life without conforming to prescriptive societal body and appearance standards. When you detach importance from culturally prescribed body and beauty standards, you can also detach importance from your looks as a whole. That doesn't mean you shouldn't like how you look. It just means that you don't have to wrap up your self-worth in the way you look, whether you like it, hate it, or feel neutral about it on any given day. As Drs. Lexie and Lindsay Kite (2020) say, "Positive body image isn't believing your body looks good; it is knowing your body is good, regardless of how it looks."

In the Kites's research, body image resilience is developed by focusing not on whether you find your body attractive or unattractive, but rather, on the way you relate to your body. Do you relate to your body from the outside, like it's an object for other people's viewing pleasure? Or do you relate to it from within, as the person inhabiting it? Consider your body as your vehicle for moving through the world, the vessel through which you experience sight, sound, smells, and other sensory information. If you connect with your body from within, you can stop objectifying yourself—treating yourself as a series of parts or objects to consume—and instead, embrace your wholeness. Whether your body is tall, short, fat, thin, muscular, soft, hairy, freckled, black, brown, peach, wrinkly, bumpy, or any other adjective…your body is not *you*. You're a living being. While yes, you *have* a body, you also have thoughts and ideas and interests and talents and feelings and memories and pet peeves and goals and dreams! Your body is simply the container and the conduit.

When you compare yourself to someone else—whether it's your sister or friend, someone on social media, a celebrity, or even an old photo of yourself—you ultimately create suffering and disconnection. Comparing involves determining that you're either better or worse than the other person, either above or below them. How can you feel close to someone if you need to think you're better than they are? Similarly, how can you be close if you're always focused on how the other person is better than you? It's hard to be vulnerable when one side is on a pedestal. We can connect with others only if we relate to each other on an equal level of shared humanity (Neff 2015). Next time you catch yourself comparing, try shifting your thoughts to more compassionate ones. Offer the other person compassionate thoughts if you've been judging them as "below" you, and offer yourself compassion if you're feeling jealous or judging yourself as "below" them.

Developing Body Image Resilience

Consider these reflection questions to help you develop a more resilient perspective on your appearance:

- How often do you think about your body or the way you look?

- How much do your feelings about your body/ looks affect your everyday mood?

- How often do the people you spend the most time with talk about bodies or physical appearance?

- How do their comments affect your mood or the way you feel about yourself?

- How much of the media and social media you consume is focused on appearance? How does what you consume affect your relationship with your body?

Now that you've taken stock of these factors, answer these questions, using your journal or a separate piece of paper:

- What would help you spend less time treating your body as an object? What would it be like to:

  - get rid of your scale and decline to be weighed (or ask for a "blind weight") at the doctor's office;

  - look in the mirror only when necessary (for example, daily hygiene routines, or checking for food in your teeth);

  - wear clothing that fits comfortably, and get rid of anything that makes you hyperfocused on your body's shape or size;

  - focus on the memory or event that was captured when looking at photos, instead of focusing on whether you like how you look in a photo?

- What can help you connect to your body from within? Can you commit to:

  - paying attention to something pleasant that your body experiences each day; for example, a warm shower, fresh air on your face, your brain thinking as you do a puzzle, your arms wrapping around a loved one;

  - writing down one thing each day that you appreciate about your body and has nothing to do with how it looks?

- What boundaries do you need to set with people in your life? Is there anyone with whom you want to try:

  - clearly and assertively telling them not to comment on your body;

  - gently changing the subject when body-talk arises;

  - distancing yourself from the relationship?

- What boundaries do you need to set with the media you consume? Would your relationship with your body improve if you were to:

  - unfollow or mute certain social media accounts;

  - reconsider the movies and TV shows you watch the most;

  - intentionally consume content that has nothing to do with displaying bodies or physical appearance?

Whether you feel positively, negatively, or neutrally about your body, it's yours for life. If you make shifts in how you think about yourself, you can create a more nuanced and compassionate perspective toward your body, *regardless* of how it looks.

Have you ever noticed how often people (especially women and femmes) give looks-based compliments? When a group of girlfriends greet each other, it often starts with a chorus of "OMG your hair looks amazing!" and "You're looking snatched in that dress!" While it can feel great to build each other up with praise, it's also risky. By giving body-based appraisals the power to validate us, we also give them the ability to destroy us (Kite and Kite 2020). Complimenting looks (and conversely, bonding over how much you hate your looks) can reinforce the idea that thinness, beauty, or being seen as attractive are the most important things. We can inadvertently become attached to our appearance as an important part of *who we are.*

Coming up with ideas and stories about who we are is a natural part of human development, and we don't just do it with our looks—we do it with various aspects of ourselves. These ideas help us develop a stable identity. For example, I'm Paula. I'm a woman, I'm a psychologist, I'm married, I'm compassionate, I'm brunette, I'm a huge fan of the reality TV show *Survivor*, I love yellow rice, and I can hold a crow pose for about thirty seconds. These things are all true about me today, and some of them have been true my entire life. The problem is that we become so strongly attached to internalized narratives about ourselves that it's hard to recognize that they might not *always* be true, or they might not *always* be important. When we become so stuck in these stories and ideas we have about ourselves, flexibility and change can seem truly impossible.

If you're someone who has gotten a lot of validation for being thin, fit, healthy, young, or looking a certain way, those attributes can become a significant part of your identity. You might be really attached to these descriptors, to the extent that if they change, it feels scary and disconcerting. In my self-description, I mentioned being brunette—but what happens if my hair goes gray? Will I still be me? Of course! But if I'm super attached to that aspect of my identity, then without my brown hair I might not *feel* like me. Similarly, if you're attached to your identity as an athlete, a sex symbol, or anything else that might change over time, it can be difficult to tolerate and accept when those things no longer describe you—or maybe they still describe you, but they're no longer the most meaningful things about you.

Detaching from the stories and ideas you have about your appearance is key for developing body image resilience. Whether you like it or not, change is the only real constant. Everyone's looks will change as they move through life. Descriptors that apply to you today, both appearance based and otherwise, may not apply to you in five, ten, or thirty years. Recognizing that change is natural for all living beings allows you to build a sense of self that is flexible, and not dependent on permanently achieving some ideal version of yourself. After all, whether its branches are heavy with fruit or frail and barren, a tree remains the same tree it has always been. You're always *you*, no matter your physical appearance, personality traits, interests, priorities, moods, or season of life.

Since you're always you, and your appearance is only an important aspect of your identity if *you* decide that it is, you can decide to focus more on your internal values and characteristics than external appearances. Consider what matters to you today. Maybe you value being a loyal friend, a loving partner, or a dedicated employee. What does that mean to you, right now? Come back to your values for guidance, and think about behaving in ways that make you proud of yourself for who you're being, not what you look like.

Validating Beyond Looks

One way to shift your focus from the outer to the inner is to practice validating other people for deeper qualities, not looks. You can use your journal for this exercise.

Write down the names of three people you feel strong love or affection toward.

Write down some of the things you love or appreciate about each of them. (Another way to think of this: what would you miss most about each if they were no longer around? Perhaps it's their generosity, their loyalty, their sense of humor?)

Was it easy or difficult to identify the things you most appreciate them for?

Where did physical appearance factor into your feelings about each person, if at all? How important is their appearance to you?

Now, think about what someone doing this exercise would say about you. List a few things you think they would write about what they love (or would miss) about you.

Are these the things you want them to validate you for? If not, what do you want people to notice about you or remember you for? How do you want people to describe you as a person?

For the next twenty-four hours, try to give compliments and praise only for qualities and characteristics that aren't based on appearance. You might try noticing things like:

- The kindness they show to you or others
- Their warm, friendly attitude

- Their infectious energy or enthusiasm

- Their creative ideas

- Their thoughtfulness or supportiveness

- Their outlook on life

- Their sense of humor

- The way they inspire you

- How you feel when you're around them

- Any quality you admire or respect about them

- Activities you enjoy doing together or interests you share

It's possible that the first thing you notice is still related to their appearance. However, if you have a strong sense of your values, you can start to notice more of the qualities and characteristics that you find meaningful. Over time, you can start to validate people for the things that matter to you, like being supportive, flexible, or compassionate. The more you practice recognizing what you value in others, the easier it can become to appreciate deeper qualities within yourself.

If you're still convinced that people in your life want you around only because of your appearance, consider whether that belief comes from them or from you. Some people in your life might say or do things that reinforce your feelings of objectification. Those relationships might be worth exploring. This doesn't mean you should cut the person off, but rather, consider having a conversation about how their behavior makes you feel. Sometimes people are so used to focusing on appearance that they don't even realize how much they talk about it. If you continue redirecting conversations and de-emphasizing looks, it's possible they will follow suit. It's also possible you'll start getting closer with the people in your life who simply don't focus on these things, or begin to develop friendships that are centered on something unrelated to appearance.

I've never seen a tombstone that read: "Here lies Sarah. She was thin and pretty." It's a cruel irony to fixate so much on appearance while living, when what we truly value in one another is much deeper. If you're unwilling to accept your body now, when will you? In ten years, twenty, or thirty? My grandmother dieted until the day she died at ninety-three. She never learned to accept the only body she ever had. Remember, accepting something doesn't mean you like it or want it to be this way. It just means that you're not going to waste energy trying to control something that's beyond your control. Once you've accepted, you can direct your energy toward respecting and honoring your body exactly as it is.

Respecting body diversity, and all facets of human diversity, will allow you to appreciate the elements of yourself that differ from other people, and the aspects of others that are unique to them. Diversity makes us beautiful! The fact that nobody out there is *exactly* like you—even if you have an identical twin—is pretty incredible. Our differences help us thrive, each bringing our strengths and balancing each other out. The systems at large will continue to objectify, denigrate, and oppress people for differences. No amount of acceptance or resilience will single-handedly change that. Yet individual actions have influence on the collective culture. You can amplify and uplift people who are different from you, and find ways that are authentic to you to fight harmful systems. You can reclaim your power, advocate for the values you believe in, and effect change by showing up unapologetically.

It won't always be easy to stay connected to your values and perspective, as long as the surrounding culture still emphasizes appearance. But if you intentionally cultivate a sense of self based on deeper qualities and characteristics, you'll be less swayed by those pressures. If you stop participating in self-objectification (and stop objectifying others), you can shift perspective from how your body is perceived, to actually experiencing life *through* your body as a vessel. When you're living from within, it doesn't matter whether you like how your body looks or think that it's beautiful. The way you feel about your body will change regardless, sometimes even in the span of a single day!

Getting attached to an idea about how you look can create long-term suffering, just as getting too attached to any other aspect of your identity can make it hard to be flexible. Holding your identity markers loosely, not tightly, can help you view yourself as a flexible, living being. You can have an identity that is *stable* without having to be *static*. In other words, you can regularly practice self-regulation and make consistent contact with your values, yet you can still change moment to moment. You're not a robot that must operate the same way over and over based on programming. By recognizing where you tend to get stuck on identity markers or labels you have attached to yourself, you can introduce more flexibility into your self-perception. This allows you to have change and movement between aspects of your identity, personality, and values from one moment to another. In chapter 13, you'll explore other aspects of your identity you may be clinging to in ways that hurt you.

CHAPTER 13

Who Are You? Like, Really...Who Are You?

The athlete: Derek started playing soccer almost as soon as he could walk. His parents and coaches knew he was something special, and by elementary school he was playing on a competitive travel team. He went to college on a soccer scholarship, and by the time he graduated, had contributed to countless tournament wins. Everyone in his life knew him as the soccer star, but realistically, he knew his soccer career would end after college. After graduating, he got a job in software sales. He still played soccer in a recreational league on weekends, but suddenly the sport went from being 80 percent of his life and identity to simply a seasonal activity. To his surprise, Derek struggled to figure out what he even enjoyed outside of soccer. He felt like he was having an identity crisis. If he wasn't Derek the soccer star, who was he?

The vegan: All of Tracy's friends came to her for healthy recipes. In her early twenties, she became vegetarian, and a few years later, went vegan. She was passionate about veganism, spending her weekends at local farmer's markets and even starting a food blog. Soon Tracy took her veganism a step further and became a raw vegan, not eating anything that had to be cooked. Even though her whole world revolved around food, she felt perpetually hungry and fatigued. Some routine blood work showed she was deficient in several vitamins and minerals. Tracy's doctor referred her to a dietitian, who recognized her restrictive eating as orthorexia, or an obsessive preoccupation with "healthy" eating that causes more harm than good. When the dietitian recommended that she begin incorporating more foods into her diet, Tracy panicked. She had built a reputation for herself as a raw vegan. If she started eating differently, what would that mean about her?

The lawyer: Monique graduated from a top law school. At graduation, she took a picture with her diploma that became her social media profile picture for the next decade. Monique was proud of how hard she had worked to become a lawyer. She wore her long, grueling hours as a badge of honor. Eventually, she worked her way up in her firm to become a partner. When she reached this milestone, she was shocked to discover that life just went on. The work kept coming, and she kept slogging away. She was passionate about practicing law, but it was starting to feel like *Groundhog Day*. Monique began to wonder if there was more to life than this all-consuming career. She found she was craving connection—a partner and family to come home to—but she worried that to date, get married, or have kids she would have to miss out on work opportunities. Ultimately, she decided that being a lawyer mattered to her, but it wasn't the *only* part of her life that mattered to her.

The mother: Victoria poured everything into her two sons. From the moment she got pregnant with her oldest, she started reading parenting books. Her main pastime when her kids were young was researching—how to encourage language development, how to raise kids with healthy self-esteem, and how to pack the most nutritious lunches. Every year, she was involved with the school's parent-teacher association; some years, that meant two associations. She sat in the bleachers cheering for her kids at every game, from Little League to high school football. She knew she'd struggle when she became an empty nester, but never predicted just how lost she would feel. After both of her sons moved out of the house, she felt a deep sense of emptiness, completely unsure what to do with herself.

The actor: Georgia was a theater kid. She earned the lead role in every school play and went to theater camp each summer. She studied theater in college, and moved to Los Angeles when she graduated. After four years of waiting tables and going to dead-end auditions, she realized that chasing her acting dreams wasn't as glamorous as she'd imagined as a kid. She lived with four strangers in a tiny, run-down apartment, and she missed her family and friends back home. She craved financial stability and a more consistent schedule. Part of her felt like changing course meant giving up or failing to achieve her dream. She eventually moved back to her hometown, where she reconnected with several old friends and got a job at a marketing agency. Georgia soon realized that she actually was enjoying this new chapter. Now that her whole world didn't revolve around trying to make it in Hollywood, she had the freedom to develop hobbies and interests outside of acting.

Each of these stories highlights ways that people can be impacted by the identities they've created. While it's helpful and even necessary to create a stable sense of identity, your attachment to that identity can become a source of suffering. You might start thinking of your descriptors, whether a job title, role, skill, religious or political affiliation, or personality trait, as *who you are* at a deeper level, rather than simply a quality or label that describes you. That aspect of your identity then feels so important that you become fixated on maintaining it. You might "set yourself up to distort the world in order to maintain this vision of yourself" (Hayes and Smith 2005).

If you're known for being funny, you can become preoccupied with making people laugh. If you're attached to being petite, you might struggle with disordered eating or become preoccupied with your size, trying to ensure that you stay small. If you're known as the life of the party, you might put on a happy face even when you're depressed. In Tracy's case, her identity as a healthy eater became such a focal point of her life that she ignored evidence that suggested her eating habits *weren't* so healthy. For Monique, it took years of discontent before she realized she was allowed to have a life outside of being a lawyer. We accidentally lock ourselves into our identities in ways that inadvertently prevent us from expanding *beyond* that one version of ourselves, and that one moment in time.

With each passing moment, you're not the same you as you were a moment ago. Getting too attached to an aspect of your identity makes it hard to cope with change. Sometimes that change is inevitable—your body and circumstances shift with the passage of time, and you're no longer a student, an athlete, or a young person. Maybe you lose your job or go through a divorce—suddenly, you're not a manager or a spouse. Other times, the change is internal—a change of heart, or a shifting of priorities or interests. You might discover that you're no longer satisfied with your job, you're no longer into playing poker, or you're no longer as devoutly religious as you previously were. Clinging tightly to an aspect of your identity can deprive you of the ability to act authentically from moment to moment.

Think back on your own history. Were there things that were big parts of your identity as a kid or teenager that aren't such an integral piece of you now? Have you discovered new interests or aspects of your personality over the years? Georgia went through this process when she decided to stop pursuing acting. Though she had mixed feelings about the change, she soon discovered that letting go of this part of her identity gave her freedom to discover new parts of herself. Not everyone has such an easy time adjusting. If you've come to identify strongly with certain markers, change can feel destabilizing, as Derek experienced when he was no longer a soccer star and Victoria struggled with when she became an empty nester.

This destabilizing experience can even happen when the aspect of identity is an unpleasant or undesired one. I notice this with clients who are so used to being anxious or depressed, or having an eating disorder that letting go of the diagnosis feels uprooting. When you're so used to identifying as anxious, or clinging to the idea that you're just depressed, it becomes difficult to recognize times when you deviate from those experiences, that you're a person who sometimes *isn't* anxious or depressed. Meanwhile, approaches like Alcoholics Anonymous and other 12-step recovery programs encourage participants to stay connected to an identity as an alcoholic or an addict, even when substance use is no longer the central part of their life. In these communities, the goal is to keep it front and center on purpose, so that the person in recovery doesn't inadvertently lose sight of the consequences of returning to old behavior patterns. While this approach has helped a lot of people, maintaining this level of attachment to a label may not be helpful for everyone, particularly if you've built a life focused on and rooted in many things *beyond* your substance-use history.

Some aspects of identity are unchangeable but still flexible. For instance, I am a trauma survivor. This will always be true—it's not going to change in twenty years. Just because this might always be true, doesn't mean it always makes sense for that aspect of my identity to be front and center. Sometimes, being a trauma survivor is relevant to the context I'm in, and other times it's not. I'm always a woman, but my gender is not always the most important thing about me. I'm a psychologist, but being a psychologist is a more relevant aspect of my identity when I'm sitting in a therapy session or writing a treatment plan than when I'm out to dinner with friends. I'm each of these things, but I'm not *just* any one of these things.

The same is true for personality traits. Your qualities and characteristics can generally describe you, but getting too attached to them can make it hard to recognize that they don't *always* apply. I think of myself as a compassionate person. I strive to behave compassionately, but there are certainly times when I'm not compassionate. You might consider yourself a friendly person, but are you *always* friendly, every moment of every day, in every environment? Probably not. In ACT, these statements and ideas about yourself are called *self-conceptualizations* (Hayes and Smith 2005). Self-conceptualization can lead to rigidity and suffering. Instead of recognizing that self-conceptualizations are just thoughts and ideas you have about yourself, you might take them as constant and important truths. It becomes hard to recognize that our identities are flexible, even when the facets that comprise them are generally consistent. When we cling too tightly to any one aspect, we don't give ourselves the chance to be multidimensional: *more* than a trauma survivor, *more* than a woman, *more* than a psychologist, *more* than compassionate.

Issues of identity get tricky when they are imposed upon you by the outside world. You might not consider your race, religion, sexual orientation, gender, ability, or size to be the most meaningful or interesting part of who you are. Yet regardless of how you feel about those parts of yourself, they are infused with socially constructed meanings that might either privilege you or add barriers to your daily life. Those facets can sometimes be forced into relevancy, making it hard for you to hold them lightly. Whether it's important to me or not, being Jewish becomes an extremely relevant part of my identity when I'm confronted with implicit or explicit antisemitism. In this way, if you're constantly told that part of you is important, you might come to identify strongly with it as a matter of self-protection.

Sometimes an aspect of identity gets passed down to you across generations. My grandmother survived the Holocaust, and most of my other relatives were murdered. The generations before that were subjected to centuries of discrimination, violence, and persecution throughout Eastern Europe.

As Jewish identity is an ethnoreligion, there are complexities to it that don't fit neatly into typical identity categories discussed in the West, making it hard for non-Jews to understand. The legacy of what it means to be Jewish was instilled in me from birth, and it's one that evokes in me a wide variety of emotions and associations on any given day. These legacies can become integrated in our DNA through transgenerational transmission.

If you belong to any community that has faced violence, discrimination, or marginalization, you likely have had this experience of being told who you are. In the United States, people who are African American might carry the legacy of trauma from a history of slavery and ongoing discrimination. When the world has decided an aspect of your identity means something specific about you, and people have been complicit in stereotyping and projecting meaning onto you, it is challenging to loosen up around identity factors. We can each only know what it's like to experience the world through our own bodies, minds, and identities. Recognizing that these aspects of identity shape and affect each of us in unique and complex ways can help us challenge the assumptions we make about others based on identity factors, and expand beyond our initial assumptions.

Who Am I?

At http://www.newharbinger.com/54063, you'll find an exercise to help you explore some of your self-conceptualizations. You'll write down the first word or descriptor that pops into your mind, completing the sentence starters "I am…," and "I am a(n)…," and "I am not…" You'll read over your responses and for each, you'll consider these questions:

Has this word or label always described me?

Will this word or label always describe me, or could it change?

Is this descriptor always an important descriptor for me?

When is this descriptor not as important, relevant, or central to how I think about myself?

Does this descriptor ever affect my choices and behaviors? How?

Does this descriptor ever affect how I feel about myself? How?

Although everything you wrote may be true about you, these things may not *always* be true, nor will they *always* be the most important or relevant things about you. You may possess certain strengths, characteristics, and personality traits; fit criteria for certain diagnoses or labels; or uphold certain roles in different spheres of your life. You're more than each of these things. You're not defined by any single experience, accomplishment, feature, or descriptor.

You do not have to attach strongly to the stories your brain tells you about who you are, nor do you have to attach strongly to the stories that the outside world projects onto you about who you are. Recognizing that these descriptors are just *stories* about you provides room for flexibility, for you to be different or focus on something different from one moment to the next. You can't control whether these ideas or stories will come into your mind, just as you can't control whether any other types of thoughts enter your mind. However, you can use mindfulness skills to notice when you get stuck on them as important or true, and then use cognitive defusion to loosen their grip. Here are some ways you might defuse from a self-conceptualization:

- "My brain is telling me that I'm an athlete, but this is only one story about me."

- "I'm noticing my mind getting really entangled with the idea that I'm a mother."

- "My mind is focusing on these feelings of anxiety, which is making them seem very important. These feelings are a moment in time; they will come and go. Feelings and thoughts don't define me."

- "Wow, my mind feels very stuck on me being outgoing and is pressuring me to act outgoing even when it's not authentic. What if I am sometimes outgoing and sometimes *not* outgoing?"

By making some space around these ideas and stories, you can hold them more flexibly. You can practice operating from your *observing self*, noticing what you're thinking, feeling, and doing from moment to moment without attaching too strongly to any particular experience, and without attaching judgments to what is happening.

Consider how any given moment has a billion different things you could deem "most important" or "most meaningful." When I'm at the beach, I could be focusing on the sand in my bathing suit, the itchy sensation between my toes, the sunshine on my face, the waves ebbing and flowing, the striped umbrella next to me, the kids building a sandcastle ten feet to my left, my critical thoughts about my body, the cold can of soda in my hand, or any other number of internal or external stimuli. That's not to say I have a choice in what I'm automatically pulled toward—usually our minds pull us toward whatever is loudest, brightest, or most unpleasant. Because our minds pull us to that detail or stimulus, it can seem like it's the most important or meaningful thing. Yet something is only an important or attention-worthy element of the moment if *you* deem it as such.

Just as you can't stop yourself from getting attached to stories, ideas, or labels, you also can't stop other people from attaching stories or labels to you. But while the world may try to tell you who you are or impose a particular set of identity markers on you, ultimately the decision to stay attached to any part of that story is up to you. Only you get to decide whether a certain story or idea about you is accurate, relevant, or meaningful. Additionally, if you practice this flexible observer attitude, you can lead by example. Instead of making assumptions about others based on one piece of information or one moment in time, you can challenge your biases and first impressions. We all get stuck on stories about who we are and who others are, but with practice we can hold these impressions and ideas more lightly.

Navigating Disruptions to Your Sense of Self

We all change. Clinging too tightly to an aspect of yourself that was once relevant or meaningful can make it hard to recognize when it no longer resonates. Some people absorb the idea that letting go of an old pursuit is quitting or giving up. Georgia worried that if she left Los Angeles, she was giving up on becoming an actor. Once she made the change, she realized she was happier moving on than clinging to a dream that was no longer authentically hers. Experiencing a shifting of priorities as you move through life is not giving up.

Similarly, you might have learned to see certain changes as signs of failure or letting yourself go. Wellness culture frames age-related changes and weight gain as failure. Hustle culture frames any slowing down or losing steam for work-related pursuits as laziness or a loss of discipline. Some common ways humans experience change are through growing older and entering a new decade, no longer being a student, getting a new job, losing a job, getting into a relationship, going through a breakup, having a child, going through different life stages with a child, encountering health problems, experiencing body changes, or aging. It is natural to go through an adjustment process when you enter a new phase of life or reach a new milestone. Encountering change is unavoidable, and not at all a sign of failure. If anything, it is a sign of being alive!

Just like you go through a grieving process when someone you love passes away, you may also go through a grieving process when you "lose" an aspect of your identity. You may sometimes find yourself nostalgic for how things used to be, or even rage against an unwanted reality. Give yourself compassion when these feelings arise. If you let yourself properly grieve— that is, acknowledge feelings of resistance, sadness, anger, and so forth, and make space for them to run their course—you may find that you eventually spend more of your time in a place of acceptance. Letting yourself properly grieve can even allow you to acknowledge something meaningful about your current season, or open up to the possibilities that may lie ahead. Humans are capable of experiencing multiple thoughts and emotions at once. You can feel sad about change, while also making space for its inevitability.

Remember that it's risky to get too attached to any aspect of identity, especially if it's one that you've come to view as your ticket to validation or belongingness. If you're used to being validated for your looks, body, or job title, it can feel devastating for those things to change. But you're bigger than any story about yourself. This is why self-compassion is more meaningful than self-esteem. According to psychologist Kristin Neff (2015), self-esteem is finicky. It can shatter with one mistake or piece of criticism. Self-compassion—the attitude of being kind to yourself simply because you exist and all living beings deserve kindness—is an approach that you can stay grounded in regardless of how smart, successful, or talented you feel in a given moment.

Your features will change, different aspects of your personality will come to the forefront at different times, and the things that serve as sources of meaning in one moment may not be that important to you at another moment. In holding your identity markers and stories about yourself lightly, you have the power to be flexible moment to moment. You can observe what you're thinking and feeling, and what's going on around you without letting it control you or mean anything about you. You're not your thoughts, feelings, personality, or looks. You're not your race, ethnicity, gender, age, shape, or size. You're not your job title, role in the family, hobbies, or interests. You're not even your values, though when you contact them regularly you might find they enhance your life. You may at times be described by some of these things, but at the end of it all, you're just *you*. A living, breathing, constantly evolving organism.

Sometimes, we unwittingly uphold the status quo even when it doesn't serve us. Now that you're familiar with your values, you're likely also more aware of just how many ways the outside world will try to pressure you to deviate from them. The culture around you might encourage you to stay stuck in stories, or make it seem like you're not supposed to change. It can be challenging to stay connected to your inner wisdom in a world that constantly urges you to ignore it. Whether through media messages, or experiences of systemic oppression, criticism, or judgment from friends and family, you'll face expectations to strive. Likewise, in your own inner world, you might face self-critical thoughts, depression, anxiety, or other internal experiences that make it challenging to stay connected to what you know is best for you. There will be no shortage of opportunities to hop back on that hamster wheel and focus on performing. It may be tempting to fall once again for those false promises that if you work harder, stay disciplined, you'll eventually reach "good enough." You can use the fluidity of identity that you have developed here to help you stay connected to your experience in any given moment.

In chapter 14, we'll tie together all the tools, skills, and wisdom you've developed throughout this book so that you can go forward confidently upon the solid foundation you've built. You now know how to defuse from unhelpful thoughts and beliefs, connect with signals from your body regarding what you need and desire, honor your values, set and maintain effective boundaries, and practice resilience and self-compassion both for disruptions to your perception of your body and your sense of self. All this awareness can help you navigate the challenges, both internal and external, that might threaten to silence your truth. You now know that you always have the option to turn inward for guidance, even when the world around you tries to convince you otherwise.

CHAPTER 14

Staying Connected to Your Truth

You may be rock solid in your values and extremely clear about what makes life meaningful to you. Still, you'll have to contend with the realities of being a person in the world. This includes facing constant pressures and influences from outside—the surrounding culture—and from within—your inner critic, old beliefs, and difficult emotions. In the world around you, you may continue to face the realities of systemic oppression, toxic media messages, and the judgment and criticism of others. In your relationships, you might have difficulty maintaining boundaries and demonstrating self-respect, especially if you still have to interact with people who expect you to behave with passive compliance.

Even with the best of intentions, you may sometimes feel pressure to chase the next accolade, follow the latest wellness trend, and fixate once again on societal expectations. You might buy into the idea that you're not supposed to change unless it's through hustle- or wellness-approved "self-improvement" efforts, so you can change as long as you're becoming more productive, wealthier, healthier, or more beautiful (but don't become *too* productive, successful or attractive because that would make you intimidating and unlikable). You'll also still experience intrusive thoughts, negative body image, self-criticism, and attachment to the stories that your brain is telling you.

These micro- and macro-level challenges can put you at risk of self-censorship. London-based consultant and writer Africa Brooke (2023) describes self-censorship as the process of excessively monitoring and silencing your true thoughts and feelings out of fear of judgment or misinterpretation. Many people engage in self-censorship thanks to cancel culture, in which people publicly pile onto an individual for not saying or doing what the group has deemed acceptable. Fear of social judgment or rejection can be so strong that it causes you to parrot whatever opinions you believe will garner approval and, thus, help you feel safe.

Self-censorship can lead to unintended consequences for your health, mental health, well-being, and ability to engage authentically in your daily life. By now you have done a deep dive into the ways that self-censorship, self-silencing, and all forms of self-denial have prevented you from enjoying your life. Even with this understanding, it is natural to want to be accepted, and to garner the approval and validation of others. Yet it is important to consider whether it serves you to follow the crowd in a given situation. It won't be easy to stay authentic when your authenticity goes against the status quo. When you feel pressure to match the opinions and beliefs of those around you, you may need to remind yourself of what you'd be giving up if you went along with their agenda.

Allie's experience, which you've read about throughout this book, can help illustrate how some of these external pressures can serve as obstacles to living intuitively or tempt you back into self-denial. A few years into her journey of healing from toxic striving, Allie found her life much more fulfilling. She was no longer fixated on looking the part of a high-powered career woman. Instead of spending exorbitant time polishing her appearance each morning, she typically threw on a casual shirt and jeans. Her office was next to a predominantly Latino high school. One afternoon, while Allie was on her way to pick up lunch, a white administrator from the school yelled out to her, assuming she was a student, and chastised her to get back to class. For a moment, Allie felt ashamed for not being clearly identifiable as a professional, and blamed herself. Then she realized that her shame came from internalized racism; being a woman of color, she was often held to higher standards of what constituted professionalism compared to her white colleagues. Many of them wore jeans all the time and were never mistaken for teens cutting class.

Allie sighed, texted her cousin to vent, and then continued toward the restaurant. When she arrived, she noticed a poster on the door advertising the restaurant's new line of "low guilt" menu items. The ad featured a thin white woman, smiling into her low-carb salad bowl. When Allie reached the front of the line, the cashier asked if she wanted to order an item from the new line. For a moment, Allie felt like she should choose the salad and forgo the club sandwich she'd been craving all morning. She took a breath and chose to honor her hunger, ordering the meal she knew would be satisfying.

Back at the office, Allie scrolled through social media before getting back to work. Even though she'd already unfollowed most of the accounts that promoted toxic messaging, today she was confronted with post after post that elicited feelings of inadequacy. First, the influencer with the perfectly decorated home office, showing off her new desk setup that promised optimal productivity. Next, a wellness account that Allie thought she'd muted beckoned her to try sprinkling a supergreen powder on her morning oatmeal for energy. She put down her phone as a male coworker approached. He asked her to send him a set of reports that Allie knew would take her an hour of tedious labor to compile. Her coworker was perfectly capable of creating the reports himself but was in the habit of coming to Allie with a helpless expression to sweet-talk her into doing tasks he found boring.

Even though Allie had a clear sense of her personal values and was committed to honoring them, she encountered daily pressures from the outside world that threatened to pull her away. Luckily, she had learned to rely on the awareness she'd developed of her bodily signals, emotions, and intuition to guide her. She was able to regularly notice when her body or mind alerted her of a discrepancy between what would be authentic to her, and what would satisfy the dominant culture. She noticed when she was being targeted by toxic messaging and did a gut check before moving forward. She noticed when she felt disrespected, and this clued her in to the need to set a boundary. She noticed when she felt overwhelmed and knew this indicated a need for some grounding and self-regulation.

Allie was constantly reminded of her inability to control other people—what they said, did, felt, or believed. Sometimes, intentionally or unintentionally, other people harmed her. They judged her and made assumptions based on her race, gender, age, clothing, and body size. Although she couldn't control how others acted, she was in charge of her own actions. She chose to attach more importance to her friends and loved ones, who had earned her respect through a track record of behaving with respect. She chose to attach less importance to the opinions of strangers, people who didn't know her well, and people who had demonstrated that their values didn't align with hers. Although she was still affected by the unfairness of the world and still felt disheartened and hopeless sometimes, she found it helpful to shift her energy toward the things she could control, and live a life of meaning and purpose in spite of these harsh realities.

Identifying External Pressures to Strive

Like Allie, you'll continue to encounter pressures, judgments, and hurtful behaviors from the people and systems around you. Knowing it's pretty much guaranteed that you'll face obstacles as you move through the world, you can reflect on the insights and skills you've developed to effectively navigate them. Take some time to consider whether you've encountered any such situations in the last few weeks. If nothing comes to mind, try to identify some of the challenging messages or situations that you're likely to encounter at some point in the future.

At http://www.newharbinger.com/54063, you'll find a series of questions that can help you identify external pressures to thrive. If you prefer, you can respond in your journal.

Where have I recently encountered unhelpful messaging trying to influence what I care about?

What can help me stay connected to my values in this type of situation?

What is realistically within my control that can help me cope when I encounter these messages?

Who in my life could be promoting toxic messaging?

What can help me stay connected to my values in this type of situation?

How can I set some boundaries with this person (either through assertive communication, changing how I interact with them, or by choosing in my own inner world to deem their input less valuable)?

Where have I been treated disrespectfully (or where do I anticipate this happening)?

What can help me stay connected to my values in this type of situation?

What is within my control that will help me navigate these experiences? Are there people or communities that can support me and help me feel empowered in the face of these experiences?

It's possible that over the course of your lifetime, systems will shift and society will progress in a different direction. It would be fantastic if you could reap the rewards of a collective effort to reject toxic striving. In the meantime, you can be part of that change. By focusing your energy on living your values, setting boundaries, and disengaging from harmful influences, you can stay connected to your truth. Your daily choices will help you build resilience in a world of pressures to strive. Don't underestimate the power you possess just by showing up in your daily life in an authentic and unapologetic way. Your actions and choices help others see what's possible. I can think of several people who inspire me by how unapologetically they live their lives, and I'm sure you can too. We learn from each other every day. Your own behavior and perspectives may have a ripple effect on the people around you, and maybe even the people around them, reaching further out into the world than you might ever know.

To stay the course, it is important to unpack not only the potential challenges from the world around you but also the disruptions that will come from within your own mind or emotions. Tanya's healing process illustrates how someone can learn to navigate inner obstacles like old beliefs, intrusive thoughts, and difficult emotions when they pop up. Over the course of her recovery process, Tanya's relationship with food and her body had transformed radically. Her actual body looked pretty much the same as it had her entire adult life, but her feelings about it were much more neutral. More importantly, the amount of time and energy she spent thinking about her body had significantly decreased. She no longer counted calories or applied rigid food rules during the week, and as a result she no longer binged on weekends.

As she became more intuitive with eating and other aspects of her life, Tanya's perspective broadened. She had mental space for other things now that she wasn't so preoccupied with doing what she was conditioned to do—going above and beyond to appeal to others and meticulously controlling her body. She discovered new interests. She joined a book club and a trivia team, and even took up knitting. With a newfound awareness of her inner needs, she was speaking up more in her relationships and setting boundaries at work. She and her boyfriend went through some growing pains while he adjusted to her increased assertiveness. He wasn't used to hearing her opinions, but ultimately, he realized he wanted to know how she felt. Their relationship deepened. At work, she was no longer in the habit of automatically saying yes when asked a favor. As a result, she was less resentful and burned out.

While she felt more satisfied with her life as a whole, Tanya still struggled with negative body image and self-critical thoughts almost daily. When she noticed her jeans getting tight, her first thought was not *Oh, I guess my body changed; it happens!* Her first thought was *Ugh, I should throw away those chips in my pantry and start tracking my food again.* When she visited her cousins, she still found herself comparing what she ordered at dinner to what they were eating.

She promoted body image resilience at work and with her friends. Because she now had the reputation of being size-inclusive, she felt an added layer of guilt when fatphobic thoughts crept in. She also continued to struggle with the belief that she should be agreeable and compliant, even at her own expense. When she said no to a request at work and a coworker pouted, she would sometimes panic and worry that she did something wrong. She'd sometimes lay in bed at night ruminating on whether a coworker hated her. All of these inner experiences of self-doubt made it hard for Tanya to trust her gut for guidance.

Tanya learned that in these moments she could rely on self-compassion, cognitive defusion, and mindfulness to get her through. She practiced noticing when her mind was stuck on a rule, like *I shouldn't eat carbs* or *I should take that extra shift.* When she noticed rigid thoughts, she tried to shift to more compassionate language. She began talking back to her inner critic, and acknowledging her thoughts with the attitude of a neutral observer. She often reminded herself that even though her brain was telling her she needed to lose weight, her brain did not always provide the most helpful ideas. When she revisited her values, she knew that returning to calorie counting was not the answer, and that her feelings about her body would come and go regardless of whether she attempted to change her size.

She gave herself compassion for sometimes grappling with fatphobia; after all, she'd lived a lifetime absorbing fatphobic messages. She didn't truly buy into those beliefs deep down, and the best she could do was to continue uncovering and unlearning her biases.

She also practiced detaching from the stories her mind told her about who she was. She had gotten attached to the idea of being a go-getter at work, so when she declined taking on extra work, she'd get scared that this meant something about her identity. With a mindful pause, she could recognize that she was a whole person. Sometimes that person stayed late, and at other times that person went home. Sometimes that person wore one clothing size, and at other times that person wore a different size. Sometimes work was at the forefront of her priorities, and at other times she was focused on spending time with her boyfriend or relaxing. She was allowed to move and change with each passing moment.

Like Tanya, you may find that your mind continues chiming in with pressures to return to old conditioning. You may also notice that your mind protests when you deviate from a story it had attached to. Intrusive and self-critical thoughts are simply parts of being alive. They might pop up from time to time, or they might pop up pretty frequently. Your goal is not to get rid of those thoughts or prevent them from arising. That would be a futile endeavor. Instead, you can work on responding to those thoughts without letting them jerk you around. Now that you can spot the red flags of a rule, you can get in the habit of recognizing when old rules pop into your head. Now that you have the option of defusing from your thoughts and treating them simply as words in your mind, you can detach importance from those ideas.

Identifying Internal Pressures to Strive

At http://www.newharbinger.com/54063, you'll find another series of questions that can help you identify pressures to thrive; this time you'll be thinking about internal pressures. If you prefer, you can respond in your journal.

Take a moment to consider some of the internal obstacles—the intrusive and self-critical thoughts, or the internal pressures to do what you've been conditioned to do—that might show up most in your life. You can treat this as a daily practice if you'd like. At the end of the day, or anytime you're feeling stuck in self-criticism, briefly reflect on the following:

What rules or ideas is my mind feeding me right now?

Where do those rules and ideas come from?

What tool(s) can help me make some space around these thoughts or feelings?

How would I respond to a friend or loved one who was struggling with self-criticism or judging themself harshly?

Assuming I might encounter this thought or judgment again, how would I like to handle it in the future?

It can be challenging to stay connected to your inner wisdom in a world that constantly urges you to ignore it. You'll face various combinations of external pressures and internal pressures, all trying to get you to go back to toxic striving. When you're surrounded by a revolving door of health, fitness, and productivity trends, it's easy to internalize the belief that you should be able to do it all without burning out. Some of us are more vulnerable to the influences of wellness and hustle cultures thanks to that interplay of nature and nurture factors—our natural personality dynamics and our experiences of being taught that we should ignore our inner signals. You may have learned to behave in ways that prioritize pleasing others over pleasing yourself.

The dominant culture promotes willpower, discipline, and self-deprivation as the keys to success, and provides privilege and reward to those who play by the rules. You might think that discipline and sacrifice are the keys to a happy life because that's what these systems teach. Unfortunately, when you turn to the outside world for instructions on how to be, you'll typically end up feeling empty and inadequate. You know by now that you can move away from this exhausting chase. You can shift your perspective from seeing yourself as the problem, to seeing impossible standards as the problem. Discipline and sacrifice aren't the only values worth upholding, especially if they lock you into a never-ending chase for a moving target. If a certain set of values ensures that you never feel attractive enough, smart enough, likable enough, or successful enough to enjoy your life, does it serve you to honor those values? Remember that you're allowed to live a rewarding and fulfilling life, just like anyone else.

Don't forget the truth those who uphold toxic systems don't want you to know: no matter how hard you work, you cannot control what you feel inside. All humans will inevitably face pain. This is true whether or not you're crushing it by societal standards. By practicing acceptance of the aspects of life that you cannot control, you can free up your energy and resources to devote to engaging in committed, values-aligned actions. You can make space unconditionally for your physical, mental, and emotional experiences, and even use those experiences as valuable sources of information about what you crave, what satisfies you, and what adds meaning and purpose to your life. When you listen to your body, you tune in to hunger, fullness, cravings, and the physiological sensations that indicate strong emotions or unmet needs. When you pay attention to your mind, you can work on challenging mental rules, detaching from your labels, and defusing from self-critical thoughts. When you attune to your emotions, you can identify feelings nonjudgmentally and treat them as messengers or alert systems, sometimes showing up to provide meaningful information. By integrating all these sources of information, you learn to live from a place of intuition.

One of my favorite reminders for my clients is that the more tools you have in your toolkit, the more flexible you can be. Having options for navigating difficult moments and situations will allow you to choose intentionally based on whatever is available to you, and whatever a given moment calls for. Your toolkit now contains important skills for cognitive defusion, boundary setting, assertive communication, interoceptive awareness, recognition of your emotions and needs, understanding of your values, commitment to acting on those values, detachment from self-conceptualizations, capacity for body image resilience, mindfulness skills, and the ability to practice self-compassion. When in doubt, you can rely on any one of these tools, or any combination thereof, integrating them in whatever ways make the most sense for you. These tools will bring you back into yourself and serve to remind you that you're the only expert on your life.

Look Within Yourself

There will always be people out there ready to tell you who to be and what to care about. Although these influences may still affect you, you now have a deeper understanding of yourself and your values. You now have the ability to tap into your intuition when you face these daily crossroads. It's up to you to think critically about what they're selling you and decide how you wish to respond. Just as there is no such thing as being a "perfect" intuitive eater, there is no such thing as being "perfectly" authentic. You're not the same exact person as you were a moment ago, and therefore what is authentic to you may shift and move in each new moment. There is no final destination to achieve; there is no need to perform. When you're feeling lost or stuck, remember to listen to your inner signals. All you can do is come back to yourself, over and over, and tune inward for information. The answers are within you; you only have to listen.

Conclusion: Thriving, Not Striving

I wrote this book for people like me—high achievers, people pleasers, and perfectionists. People who are constantly striving, but never feel like they're reaching a destination worth being proud of. Lots of us have a natural inclination toward striving, which could be channeled effectively into an adaptive form of perfectionism. In many situations, a conscientious personality and a strong desire to work toward goals can serve as assets. But when the outside world preys on these tendencies and conditions us to chase validation and approval, our natural inclinations get stoked into an all-consuming bonfire of self-torture. We develop a pattern of striving that is toxic to our minds and bodies. We focus on seeking impossible standards, instead of turning inward for guidance on what makes life meaningful.

I had a high school teacher who used to say "Maybe instead of pointing the finger, you should be pulling back the thumb." While writing this book, I had a lot of "pull back the thumb" moments where I caught myself chasing hustle and wellness ideals. Last summer, we had to put our dog to sleep the same week I was onboarding a new group of interns to my practice. My automatic response was not to attend to my needs and act authentically, but rather to try to tamp down my grief so I could do my job with a smile. Eventually I remembered to pause, breathe, and model the same vulnerability I ask my students to bring to their work. Shortly thereafter, I gained some weight during back-to-back IVF cycles and had to go up a few sizes. My immediate reaction was panic, and an urge to avoid an upcoming event because I hated how I looked in my dress. It took an intense therapy session, some journaling, and a lot of cognitive defusion to make space for those feelings. I had to intentionally detach meaning from my appearance, instead of raging against my body or engaging in behaviors that went against my values.

Sometimes, being well equipped to teach others these lessons while struggling to apply them to myself can make me feel like a fraud. Despite spending my days helping people break free from these pressures, I still get hit with life's curveballs, just like anyone else. I still struggle with thoughts that I'm not doing enough, that I'm lazy and selfish. I still find myself plagued by the belief that I should be less opinionated, more agreeable, and more compliant. I still get tempted to look for life hacks and shortcuts to optimize my functioning. I still get enticed by the illusion that full control is possible if I could just harness some discipline and willpower.

These intrusive thoughts, uncomfortable feelings, and pressures to strive may simply be par for the course after a lifetime of absorbing messages from wellness and hustle cultures. I know deep down that they don't make me a phony—they just make me human! The best I can do is notice them, name them, and gently challenge them. If we get too stuck on needing to be perfectly free from critical thoughts, perfectly detached from unhelpful beliefs, perfectly intuitive with how we eat, perfectly values aligned with how we behave, or perfectly mindful and present in our lives, then we're just transferring our striving efforts to a new set of unrealistic standards. As my friend Jenna Jozefowski often says, it's easy to fall for "another flavor of the same sh*t sandwich."

Even if, like me, you're steadily committed to your own path, you'll probably also grapple with unwanted thoughts and feelings, or temptations to just do what society expects. There will be pain no matter what, because pain is a natural part of being alive. There is pain in staying trapped in the chase. There is also pain in leaving it behind, and with it, the illusion of achieving pure happiness. Since there is no pain-free option, you might as well choose the pain that leads you in the direction of greater meaning. Striving to satisfy the outside world can keep you on a road to nowhere, while moving in the direction of your own inner compass will take you down a path of purpose and true well-being. Only you can decide which road to choose at any given moment.

No matter how much resilience you build, and no matter how much healing you experience, you'll likely grow faster than the systems around you. Progress happens in fits and starts, over years and years. In the meantime, these unfair systems will continue to privilege people who fit the mold and stigmatize people who don't. It's understandable if it's hard to navigate this reality. There may always be a part of you that wants to conform in order to get privilege or validation and have an easier time moving through the world. Giving up the chase for privilege can sometimes mean accepting more pain or difficulties, and it's okay if that's a complicated choice for you. When possible, surrounding yourself with a values-aligned community can help embolden you to keep honoring your values over those of wellness and hustle cultures. Your decisions have a ripple effect on the people around you, and living from your values can attract others toward you who share those values.

Even if you've decided to opt out, you can't completely rid yourself of toxic messaging. You may continue to find tendrils of wellness and hustle cultures wrapping around parts of your psyche that you thought you'd unearthed. Luckily, you've become intimately familiar with your body, mind, and emotions. You can recognize when you're honoring your needs and when you're denying or ignoring your truth. Continuing to flex those attunement muscles will help you notice signs that you're slipping back into a rigid or perfectionistic mindset.

Taking up space and pursuing things that bring you pleasure or satisfaction may still feel foreign. If you were taught that your needs shouldn't be prioritized, or made to feel responsible for ensuring the emotional comfort of people around you, it might take a while to get used to tapping into your needs. It might still feel safer to act in ways that are accommodating or pleasing, even if those behaviors go against your true wishes and desires. If you slip back into patterns of denying your needs to placate others, don't treat this as a sign of backsliding. Instead, try to get curious about what's happening. Perhaps you'll realize you need to set some boundaries, or perhaps you'll simply discover an opportunity to offer yourself compassion.

Even when you're feeling secure, the toxicity of the outside world might threaten to pull you back in. I wish you never had to face those pressures, but unfortunately they will continue to rear their ugly heads. The outside world is not within your control. However, you're not powerless. You have control over your responses to messages from both your own mind and the outside world. You choose how you respond to negative or self-critical thoughts when they pop up—and of course they will pop up! You choose how you cope with difficult emotions. You can't control whether your attention gets hijacked or whether you become distracted, but you have control over redirecting yourself when this happens. You have the ability to intentionally direct your focus toward meaningful topics or stimuli. You choose which relationships you invest energy into, and where you set boundaries. You decide how you consume media and social media. You're in charge of how you behave as you move through life, how you treat other people, how you treat yourself, what you say, and how you say it.

If you're prone to chasing accolades and striving to meet unattainable standards, you can easily turn anything into a chase. But as my own therapist taught me many years ago, intuition can't be chased. It makes itself known when you turn inward and make space for it. Try to be patient and gentle with yourself, as there is no such thing as being perfectly attuned, assertive, or expressive. You can't force your intuition to show itself, but you can cultivate a fertile ground as you wait for it to sprout. You can practice regularly integrating information from your mind, body, emotions, and personal values. Notice when you're experiencing a strong need—whether for something physical like food or sleep, or something psychological and emotional, like connection, creative expression, or feeling seen and heard. Notice your gut instincts; they'll give you a sense of when something feels right or when it seems off. Don't forget that your sensations and emotions can sometimes (but not always!) bring valuable messages about your true desires and unmet needs. Opening up to your physical and emotional worlds will provide you with the chance to listen to these messages, and over time your intuition will show up more clearly.

When in doubt, come back to your values. They will steer you to behave in ways that make you proud of yourself. Following your values and validating yourself for the deeper qualities you strive to embody will help you break away from performing for the approval of others. Although you'll still contend with the pressures of toxic striving that swirl both around you and within you, you can live freely, less susceptible to their influence. You can now tell the difference between your own true path and the expectations you were conditioned to care about. You have a choice, and in this choice lies your power. You have the power to honor your own well-being and quality of life. You need not waste any more of your precious time on this planet striving for toxic standards.

Acknowledgments

I'll never forget the day I first learned about acceptance and commitment therapy. Sitting in class, I thought to myself, *Okay, this makes sense!* ACT quickly became my favorite way to practice psychotherapy, especially with anxious strivers who struggle to tolerate imperfection. Thank you to all of the ACT scholars and theorists who have shaped my understanding of the framework: Steven Hayes, Russ Harris, Robyn Walser, Kirk Strosahl, and Jason Luoma, to name a few. Thank you to my ACT-loving colleagues, supervisors, and friends who have inspired me to apply the theory in unique ways over the years: Heather Oleson, Kirstin Quinn Siegel, Sarah Pegrum, Sari Ticker, Savana Howe, Jenny Sokolowski—and I could never forget the OG, Uri Heller.

My work got a million times deeper when I discovered the intuitive eating model and became a size-inclusive clinician. Evelyn Tribole, Elyse Resch, Christy Harrison, Lisa DuBrueil, Sabrina Strings, Maria Paredes, Jessamyn Stanley, Judith Matz, Sonya Renee Taylor, Jennifer Gaudiani, Lexie Kite, and Lindsay Kite have profoundly influenced my understanding of food and body struggles and the cultural forces that uphold them. My friend and colleague Jenna Jozefowski helped me think critically about how any framework can become cultish, even the ones that push back against toxic systems.

This book has been brewing in me for several years, until a fortuitous chain of events at the 2022 ACBS World Conference gave me an opening to share it with the world. Thank you to Erin Heath for your insight on pitching to publishers and for introducing me to Elizabeth Hollis Hansen, who saw the potential in this book and stuck with me as we polished the idea. Thank you to Elizabeth, Callie Brown, and the team at New Harbinger Publications for coming up with the phrase *"toxic striving"* to describe this all-too-familiar struggle. Thank you to Jenny Sokolowski for your valuable insight throughout the manuscript writing. Thank you to Sari Ticker and Alissa Schor for your input on those early chapters.

Jenny Sokolowski and Hannah Pavett, you bring the vibes to HumanKind Psych. Your wit, energy, humor, and warmth are what make our team thrive. Thank you to my student trainees, past, present, and future, for your willingness to grow alongside me and for reminding me how cool this work is.

I did not expect to be writing my dream book while undergoing multiple rounds of fertility treatment, but life is messy. I wrote most of this manuscript in the waiting room at Fertility Centers of Illinois. Thank you to my IVF friends who taught me how to give myself grace on the days I just couldn't wear my clinician hat, and when the hormones had me convinced every word I wrote was garbage. Jordan Roddey and Diana Siew, you're so wise, powerful, and resilient. Worst club, best members.

Behind every great therapist is a great therapist. Chris, you're it. You connected me to my intuition and trusted my wisdom before I even knew it was in there.

To my beautiful family: Donna and Joel Freedman, Dara, Adam, and Sarah, and the best in-laws a gal could ask for—Judi and Steven Diamond, Justin, Amy, Jordan, and Kasey. To my nieces Harper and Sadie, may you grow up surrounded by a culture that honors all differences, and never feel pressure to strive toward arbitrary standards. To my incredible grandmother, Shelly Weiner, you have been my lifelong role model in authenticity and acceptance. To the sweetest puggle, Kramer: I miss my writing buddy every day.

To my bestie, *bashert*, and beloved, Jeremy David: thank you for fueling my ambition, encouraging me to take chances, talking about feelings more regularly than you might prefer, and brainstorming ideas for books and business ventures. Lastly, to my baby: I love you with every cell in my body.

Additional Resources

Gaudiani, J. 2018. *Sick Enough: A Guide to the Medical Complications of Eating Disorders*, 1st ed. New York: Routledge.

Luoma, J. B., S. C. Hayes, and R. D. Walser. 2007. *Learning ACT: An Acceptance and Commitment Therapy Skills Training Manual for Therapists*. Oakland, CA: New Harbinger Publications.

Matz, J., and E. Frankel. 2024. *Beyond a Shadow of a Diet: The Comprehensive Guide to Treating Binge Eating Disorder, Emotional Eating, and Chronic Dieting*, 3rd ed. New York: Routledge.

Paterson, R. 2000. *The Assertiveness Workbook: How to Express Your Ideas and Stand Up for Yourself at Work and in Relationships*. Oakland, CA: New Harbinger Publications.

References

Adler, A. 2010. *What Life Should Mean to You.* George Allen & Unwin, 1932. Reprint. Eastford, CT: Martino Fine Books.

Bacon, L. 2008. *Health at Every Size: The Surprising Truth About Your Weight.* Dallas: BenBella Books.

Bacon, L., and L. Aphramor. 2011. "Weight Science: Evaluating the Evidence for a Paradigm Shift." *Nutrition Journal* 10(1): 9.

Baranek, L. K. 1996. "The Effect of Rewards and Motivation on Student Achievement." Master's thesis, Grand Valley State University, 285.

Brewerton, T. D. 2007. "Eating Disorders, Trauma, and Comorbidity: Focus on PTSD." *Eating Disorders* 15(4): 285–304.

Brooke, A. 2023. "Are You Self-Censoring? Understanding Communication Styles in Today's Culture." *Beyond the Self* (podcast), June 5. https://africabrooke.com /podcast/053-are-you-self-censoring-understanding-communication-styles-in -todays-culture.

Brown, B. 2010. "The Power of Vulnerability." *TEDxHouston*, June. https://www.ted .com/talks/brene_brown_the_power_of_vulnerability.

Brownell, K. D., and J. Rodin. 1994. "Medical, Metabolic, and Psychological Effects of Weight Cycling." *Archives of Internal Medicine* 154(12): 1325–1330.

Burgard, D. 2009. "What Is Health at Every Size?" In *The Fat Studies Reader*, edited by E. Rothblum and S. Solovay. New York: New York University Press.

Cameron, J. D., G. S. Goldfield, G. Finlayson, J. E. Blundell, and R. Doucet. 2014. "Fasting for 24 Hours Heightens Reward from Food and Food-Related Cues." *PLoS ONE* 9(1): e85970.

Cho, Y. J., and J. L. Perry. 2012. "Intrinsic Motivation and Employee Attitudes: Role of Managerial Trustworthiness, Goal Directedness, and Extrinsic Reward Expectancy." *Review of Public Personnel Administration* 32(4): 382–406.

Cobbaert, L., and A. Rose. 2023. *Eating Disorders and Neurodivergence: A Stepped Care Approach.* Eating Disorders Neurodiversity Australia (EDNA) and the National Eating Disorders Collaboration (NEDC).

Diaz, V. A., A. G. Mainous, and C. J. Everett. 2005. "The Association Between Weight Fluctuation and Mortality: Results from a Population-Based Cohort Study." *Journal of Community Health* 30(3): 153–165.

Edirisooriya, W. A. 2014. "Impact of Rewards on Employee Performance: With Special Reference to ElectriCo." *Proceedings of the 3rd International Conference on Management and Economics* 26(1): 311–318.

Epstein, L. H., R. Truesdale, A. Wojcik, R. A. Paluch, and H. A. Raynor. 2003. "Effects of Deprivation on Hedonics and Reinforcing Value of Food." *Physiology and Behavior* 78(2): 221–227.

Fothergill, E., J. Guo, L. Howard, J. C. Kerns, N. D. Knuth, R. Brychta, K. Y. Chen, et al. 2016. "Persistent Metabolic Adaptation 6 Years After The Biggest Loser Competition." *Obesity* 24(8): 1612–1619.

Grant, A. 2008. "Does Intrinsic Motivation Fuel the Prosocial Fire? Motivational Synergy in Predicting Persistence, Performance, and Productivity." *The Journal of Applied Psychology* 93: 48–58.

Hagan, M. M., and D. E. Moss. 1997. "Persistence of Binge-Eating Patterns After a History of Restriction with Intermittent Bouts of Refeeding on Palatable Food in Rats: Implications for Bulimia Nervosa." *The International Journal of Eating Disorders* 22(4): 411–420.

Haines, J., D. Neumark-Sztainer, M. Eisenberg, and P. Hannan. 2006. "Weight Teasing and Disordered Eating Behaviors in Adolescents: Longitudinal Findings From Project EAT (Eating Among Teens)." *Pediatrics* 117(2): e209–e215.

Hancock, A. 2023. "Anti-Aging Market Size, Share, Trends, Opportunities Analysis Forecast Report by 2030." Vantage Market Research.

Harrison, C. 2019. *Anti-Diet: Reclaim Your Time, Money, Well-Being, and Happiness Through Intuitive Eating*. New York: Little, Brown Spark.

———. 2023. *The Wellness Trap: Break Free from Diet Culture, Disinformation, and Dubious Diagnoses, and Find Your True Well-Being*. New York: Little, Brown Spark.

Hayes, S. C., and S. Smith. 2005. *Get Out of Your Mind and Into Your Life: The New Acceptance and Commitment Therapy*. Oakland, CA: New Harbinger Publications.

Hersey, T. 2022. *Rest Is Resistance: A Manifesto*. New York: Little, Brown Spark.

Hood, C. M., K. P. Gennuso, G. R. Swain, and B. B. Catlin. 2016. "County Health Rankings: Relationships Between Determinant Factors and Health Outcomes." *American Journal of Preventive Medicine* 50(2): 129–135.

Huddleston, C. 2019. "46% of Americans Need a Side Hustle Just to Cover Basic Expenses." *GOBankingRates*, May 20.

Istvan, E. M., R. E. Nevill, and M. O. Mazurek. 2020. "Sensory Over-Responsivity, Repetitive Behavior, and Emotional Functioning in Boys With and Without Autism Spectrum Disorder." *Research in Autism Spectrum Disorders* 75.

Jack, D. C., and D. Dill. 1992. "The Silencing the Self Scale: Schemas of Intimacy Associated with Depression in Women." *Psychology of Women Quarterly* 16(1): 97–106.

Jakubowski, K. P., E. Barinas-Mitchell, Y. F. Chang, P. M. Maki, K. A. Matthews, and R. C. Thurston. 2022. "The Cardiovascular Cost of Silence: Relationships Between Self-silencing and Carotid Atherosclerosis in Midlife Women." *Annals of Behavioral Medicine: A Publication of the Society of Behavioral Medicine* 56(3): 282–290.

Kabat-Zinn, J. 2005. *Wherever You Go, There You Are: Mindfulness Meditation in Everyday Life*. New York: Hachette Books.

———. 2013. *Full Catastrophe Living: Using the Wisdom of Your Body and Mind to Face Stress, Pain, and Illness*. New York: HarperCollins.

Kite, L., and L. Kite. 2020. *More Than a Body: Your Body Is an Instrument, Not an Ornament.* Boston: Houghton Mifflin Harcourt.

———. 2024. *Official Workbook for More Than a Body.* More Than a Body LLC.

Kutscheidt, K., T. Dresler, J. Hudak, B. Barth, F. Blume, T. Ethofer, A. J. Fallgatter, and A. C. Ehlis. 2019. "Interoceptive Awareness in Patients with Attention-Deficit/Hyperactivity Disorder (ADHD)." *Attention Deficit and Hyperactivity Disorders* 11(4): 395–401.

Lane, S. J., S. Reynolds, and L. Thacker. 2010. "Sensory Over-Responsivity and ADHD: Differentiating Using Electrodermal Responses, Cortisol, and Anxiety." *Frontiers in Integrative Neuroscience* 4: 603.

Lo, A., and M. J. Abbott. 2013. "Review of the Theoretical, Empirical, and Clinical Status of Adaptive and Maladaptive Perfectionism." *Behaviour Change* 30(2): 96–116.

López-Gil, J. F., P. J. Tárraga-López, M. S. Hershey, R. López-Bueno, H. Gutiérrez-Espinoza, A. Soler-Marín, A. Fernández-Montero, and D. Victoria-Montesinos. 2023. "Overall Proportion of Orthorexia Nervosa Symptoms: A Systematic Review and Meta-Analysis Including 30476 Individuals from 18 Countries." *Journal of Global Health* 13: 04087.

Maji, S., and S. Dixit. 2019. "Self-Silencing and Women's Health: A Review." *International Journal of Social Psychiatry* 65(1): 3–13.

Mann, T., A. J. Tomiyama, E. Westling, A. Lew, B. Samuels, and J. Chatman. 2007. "Medicare's Search for Effective Obesity Treatments: Diets Are Not the Answer." *American Psychologist* 62(3): 220–233.

Maslow, A. 1943. "A Theory of Human Motivation." *Psychological Review* 50: 370–396.

Matz, J., and E. Frankel. 2024. *Beyond a Shadow of a Diet: The Comprehensive Guide to Treating Binge Eating Disorder, Emotional Eating, and Chronic Dieting,* 3rd ed. New York: Routledge.

McGovern, L. 2014. "The Relative Contribution of Multiple Determinants to Health Outcomes." *Health Affairs,* August 21. https://www.healthaffairs.org/content/briefs/relative-contribution-multiple-determinants-health.

Miller, L. J., S. A. Schoen, S. Mulligan, and J. Sullivan. 2017. "Identification of Sensory Processing and Integration Symptom Clusters: A Preliminary Study." *Occupational Therapy International* 2017: 2876080.

Neff, K. 2015. *Self-Compassion: The Proven Power of Being Kind to Yourself.* New York: William Morrow.

Neumark-Sztainer, D., N. Falkner, M. Story, C. Perry, P. Hannan, and S. Mulert. 2002. "Weight-Teasing Among Adolescents: Correlations with Weight Status and Disordered Eating Behaviors." *International Journal of Obesity* 26(1): 123–131.

Newport, C. 2019. *Digital Minimalism: Choosing a Focused Life in a Noisy World.* New York: Penguin Random House.

Petersen, A. 2020. *Can't Even: How Millennials Became the Burnout Generation.* New York: HarperCollins.

Petrzela, N. M. 2022. *Fit Nation: The Gains and Pains of America's Exercise Obsession*. Chicago: University of Chicago Press.

Prilleltensky, I. 2019. "Mattering at the Intersection of Psychology, Philosophy, and Politics." *American Journal of Community Psychology* 65: 1–19.

Puhl, R. 2019. "Weight Discrimination Is Rampant. Yet in Most Places It's Still Legal." *Washington Post*, June 21. https://www.washingtonpost.com/outlook /weight-discrimination-is-rampant-yet-in-most-places-its-still-legal/2019/06 /21/f958613e-9394-11e9-b72d-d56510fa753e_story.html.

Puhl, R. M., and K. D. Brownell. 2006. "Confronting and Coping with Weight Stigma: An Investigation of Overweight and Obese Adults." *Obesity* 14(10): 1802–1815.

Ravenelle, A. 2019. *Hustle and Gig: Struggling and Surviving in the Sharing Economy*. Berkeley, CA: University of California Press.

Rhee, E. J. 2017. "Weight Cycling and Its Cardiometabolic Impact." *Journal of Obesity and Metabolic Syndrome* 26(4): 237–242.

Schmitt, C., and S. Schoen. 2022. "Interoception: A Multi-Sensory Foundation of Participation in Daily Life." *Frontiers in Neuroscience* 16: 875200.

Shouse, S. H., and J. Nilsson. 2011. "Self-Silencing, Emotional Awareness, and Eating Behaviors in College Women." *Psychology of Women Quarterly* 35(3): 451–457.

Strings, S. 2019. *Fearing the Black Body: The Racial Origins of Fat Phobia*. New York: New York University Press.

Taylor, J. B. 2008. *My Stroke of Insight: A Brain Scientist's Personal Journey*. New York: Penguin Random House.

Tribole, E., and E. Resch. 2020. *Intuitive Eating: A Revolutionary Anti-Diet Approach*, 4th ed. New York: St. Martin's Essentials.

Tseng, J., and J. Poppenk. 2020. "Brain Meta-State Transitions Demarcate Thoughts Across Task Contexts Exposing the Mental Noise of Trait Neuroticism." *Nature Communications* 11: 3480.

Tylka, T. L., R. A. Annunziato, D. Burgard, S. Daníelsdóttir, E. Shuman, C. Davis, and R. M. Calogero. 2014. "The Weight-Inclusive Versus Weight-Normative Approach to Health: Evaluating the Evidence for Prioritizing Well-Being over Weight Loss." *Journal of Obesity* 2014: 983495.

Ussher, J. M., and J. Perz. 2010. "Gender Differences in Self-Silencing and Psychological Distress in Informal Cancer Carers." *Psychology of Women Quarterly* 34(2): 228–242.

Wallace, J. 2023. *Never Enough: When Achievement Culture Becomes Toxic— and What We Can Do About It*. New York: Penguin Random House.

World Health Organization (WHO). 2021. "Long Working Hours Increasing Deaths from Heart Disease and Stroke: WHO, ILO." *WHO*, May 17. https:// www.who.int/news/item/17-05-2021-long-working-hours-increasing-deaths -from-heart-disease-and-stroke-who-ilo.

———. n.d. "Social Determinants of Health." Retrieved October 2023. https:// www.who.int/health-topics/social-determinants-of-health#tab=tab_1.

Paula Freedman-Diamond, PsyD, is a licensed clinical psychologist, certi-fied intuitive eating counselor, and owner and clinical director of HumanKind Psychological Services, where she specializes in treating anxiety, perfectionism, and disordered eating. She regularly contributes to *Psychology Today* in her online series, "Fat Is Not a Feeling." She has been a featured expert for *The New York Times*, *Oxygen*, *Allure*, Reebok, and Bark Technologies. She regularly provides mental-health advocacy, education, and engaging content to her audience on Instagram and TikTok.

Foreword writer **Nancy Colier, LCSW, Rev.,** is a psychotherapist, author, interfaith minister, and public speaker. She is a thought leader on mindful-ness, well-being, and digital life; and is author of *The Power of Off* and *Can't Stop Thinking.*

Real change *is* possible

For more than fifty years, New Harbinger has published proven-effective self-help books and pioneering workbooks to help readers of all ages and backgrounds improve mental health and well-being, and achieve lasting personal growth. In addition, our spirituality books offer profound guidance for deepening awareness and cultivating healing, self-discovery, and fulfillment.

Founded by psychologist Matthew McKay and Patrick Fanning, New Harbinger is proud to be an independent, employee-owned company. Our books reflect our core values of integrity, innovation, commitment, sustainability, compassion, and trust. Written by leaders in the field and recommended by therapists worldwide, New Harbinger books are practical, accessible, and provide real tools for real change.

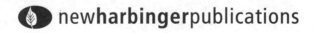 **newharbinger**publications

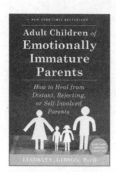
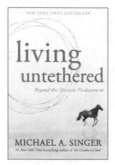
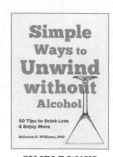
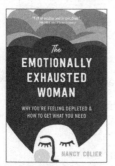
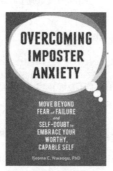
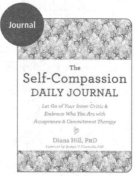